Communication
for Nurses

*How to Prevent Harmful Events
and Promote Patient Safety*

Pamela McHugh Schuster
and **Linda Nykolyn**

Communication
for **Nurses**

*How to Prevent Harmful Events
and Promote Patient Safety*

 F.A. Davis Company • Philadelphia

F. A. Davis Company
1915 Arch Street
Philadelphia, PA 19103
www.fadavis.com

Printed in the United States of America

Last digit indicates print number: 10 9 8 7 6 5 4 3 2 1

Senior Acquisitions Editor: Thomas A. Ciavarella
Director of Content Development: Darlene D. Pedersen
Project Editor: Meghan K. Ziegler
Assistant Editor: Maria Z. Price
Manager of Design and Illustration: Carolyn O'Brien

As new scientific information becomes available through basic and clinical research, recommended treatments and drug therapies undergo changes. The author(s) and publisher have done everything possible to make this book accurate, up to date, and in accord with accepted standards at the time of publication. The author(s), editors, and publisher are not responsible for errors or omissions or for consequences from application of the book, and make no warranty, expressed or implied, in regard to the contents of the book. Any practice described in this book should be applied by the reader in accordance with professional standards of care used in regard to the unique circumstances that may apply in each situation. The reader is advised always to check product information (package inserts) for changes and new information regarding dose and contraindications before administering any drug. Caution is especially urged when using new or infrequently ordered drugs.

Library of Congress Cataloging-in-Publication Data

Library of Congress Cataloging-in-Publication Data

Schuster, Pamela McHugh, 1953-
  Communication for nurses : how to prevent harmful events and promote patient safety / Pamela McHugh Schuster, Linda Nykolyn.
    p.; cm.
  Includes bibliographical references and index.
  ISBN 978-0-8036-2080-3 (pbk. : alk. paper) 1. Communication in nursing. 2. Nurse and patient. 3. Medical errors—Prevention. I. Nykolyn, Linda. II. Title.
  [DNLM: 1. Nurse-Patient Relations. 2. Communication. 3. Medical Errors—prevention & control. 4. Patient Care Management. 5. Safety Management. WY 87 S395ca 2010]
  RT23.S38 2010
  610.7306'99—dc22

                                                                                    2009044439

This book is dedicated to nurses, nursing students, and nursing faculty, who comprise the largest discipline within the health-care workforce and must keep themselves updated on the development of the latest patient-safe communication strategies to prevent harmful events to patients.

This book is also dedicated to our families, colleagues, and friends who have supported us throughout our efforts in developing this book.

Pamela McHugh Schuster

This book is dedicated to my mother Sophie, the kindest and most caring person I have ever known; and to my siblings, friends, colleagues, staff, and everyone from F.A. Davis who provided me with support and encouragement every step of the way!

Linda Nykolyn

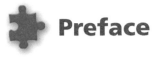 **Preface**

The purpose of this book is to guide the development of comprehensive professional communication strategies in nursing students to prevent communication errors that result in patient injuries and death. In 2000, the Institute of Medicine reported in "To Err is Human" that harmful events result in 48,000 to 98,000 deaths per year, in minutes, that amounts to 1 death every 5–10 minutes. Health-care leaders all over the world were stunned. Few could believe what they were reading. Over the past 9 years continued analysis of harmful events by the Joint Commission in the United States led to the conclusion that communication errors are the root cause of 70% of sentinel events in health-care settings. In recent years, accrediting agencies in the United States and Canada and the World Health Organization have developed goals and strategies to improve the effectiveness of communication among caregivers.

In this book, we consider communication to be the key instrument used by nurses and all health-care providers for ensuring patient safety. Health-care providers use communication in all aspects of patient care, 24 hours a day, 365 days a year. If communications fail at any point, the failure can lead to patient harm.

Unfortunately, we cannot prevent all harmful events to patients in health-care settings; but there are many ways to decrease the frequency of serious patient injuries and deaths due to misinterpretations and gaps in communication. To use communication as a patient safety instrument, you need expertise and knowledge of:

- The basic fundamentals of patient-safe communication in developing interpersonal relationships
- How to use patient-safe communication to establish effective nurse-patient relationships to ensure active participation of the patient and family in planning, implementing, and evaluating plans of care, and
- How to use patient-safe communication when collaborating with other members of the health-care team.

To assist students with attaining this expertise and knowledge, we have developed this book and Web-based ancillaries in three units.

The first unit of this book is about interpersonal communication and building the foundations for patient-safe communication. The fundamentals of how individual communication patterns are shaped by interpersonal and external factors are explored. Communication is described from various perspectives to promote self-awareness and understanding of ways to improve communication effectiveness within interpersonal relationships. The Transformational Model of Patient-Safe Communication is introduced, focused on the effects and outcomes of the communication process that are especially relevant in health-care communications.

The second unit of this book is about patient-safe communication in professional nurse-patient relationships. The developing nurse must now transition from understanding the basics of communication into using specific patient-safe communication strategies within professional nurse-patient relationships. Effective patient-safe communication strategies basic and vital to establishing and maintaining collaborative nurse-patient relationships are explored. The Patient-Safe Communication Process, derived from the Transformational Model of Communication, is introduced as a key patient-safe communication strategy for appropriate and effective communication. The third unit of this book is about health-care team communication and group processes used to promote patient-safe communication between members of the health-care team. Nurses work in multidisciplinary teams, and effective interdisciplinary communication is essential to promote patient-safe communication between members of the health-care team and to promote a culture of patient safety. An understanding of group processes is essential to facilitate effective professional communications in groups to promote optimal patient health transformational outcomes. The nursing work system and conditions in the work environment that create communication failures and harmful events are explored, and health-care team patient-safe communication strategies designed to build safety into health care and prevent patient care errors are described.

The evidence is clear: there is an astounding lack of communication in health-care settings, resulting in harmful events to patients. This book and its ancillaries will help you to develop high-level competence in communication and use patient-safe communication strategies to keep patients safe from harmful events and to build a safer health-care system.

We wish to acknowledge and thank our editors Tom Ciavarella, Meghan Ziegler, and Caryn Abramowitz for their support and encouragement throughout the writing and production of this book.

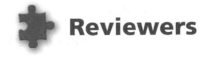

Reviewers

Kathleen Anderson, MS, RNP-C
Nurse Practitioner
Binghamton University
East Vestal, New York

Heidi Matarasso Bakerman, RN, BS, MScN
Nursing Instructor
Vanier College
St. Laurent, Quebec

Katrina Blacklock, RN, BScN, MEd
Curriculum Control Instructor
NorQuest College
Edmonton, Alberta

Stephanie Chalupka, EdD, APRN, BC, CNS, FAAAOHN
Professor and Coordinator
Worcester State College
Worcester, Massachusetts

Yvonne L. Chesna, RN, MS, FNP
Family Nurse Practitioner and Clinical
Faculty Instructor
Binghamton University
Binghamton, New York

Petrine Churchill, RN, BN
Faculty
NSCC Burridge Campus
Yarmouth, Nova Scotia

Katherine E. Cummings, BScN, MHSc, RN, RCRT
Professor
Durham College
Oshawa, Ontario

Sandra Davidson, RN, MSN, CNE
Clinical Associate Professor
Arizona State University
Phoenix, Arizona

Andrea Deakin, RN, HBScN
Coordinator
Mohawk College of Applied Arts and
Technology
Hamilton, Ontario

Sally A. Decker, PhD, RN
Professor of Nursing
Saginaw Valley State University
University Center, Michigan

Mary Elliott, RN, BScN, MEd
Professor
Humber
Toronto, Ontario

Marilyn Kelly, RN, BN, MEd
Coordinator
Conestoga College
Kitchener, Ontario

Linda Ann Kucher, MSN, RN, CMSRN
Associated Professor of Nursing
Gordon College
Barnesville, Georgia

Gail A. Mathieson-Devereaux, MS, RN, FNP-C
Clinical Instructor
Binghamton University
Binghamton, New York

Barbara Maxwell, MSN, MS, BSN, RN
Associate Professor of Nursing
SUNY Ulster
Stone Ridge, New York

Carrie Mines, RN, BScN, MSc(T), PhD
Faculty
Mohawk College
Hamilton, Ontario

Denise Newton-Mathur, RN, BA
Lecturer
Laurentian University
Sudbury, Ontario

Cindy Noble, RN, BNSc, MN, PNC(c)
Professor
Sheridan Institute of Technology and
    Advanced Learning
Brampton, Ontario

Linda O'Halloran, BScN, MScN, RN
Nursing Professor
St. Clair College of Applied Arts and
    Technology
Chatham, Ontario

Jason Powell, RN, BScN, MScN, PhD
Chair for Nursing Programs
Conestoga Institute of Technology and
    Advanced Learning
Kitchener, Ontario

Leata Rigg, RegN, BScN, MN
Professor
Nothern College of Applied Arts and
    Technology
Timmins, Ontario

Linda E. Reese, RN, BS, MA
Associate Professor
College of Staten Island
Staten Island, New York

Elizabeth Roe, RN PhD
Associated Professor of Nursing
Saginaw Valley State University
University Center, Michigan

Cheryl S. Sadler, BSN, MEd, MSN, PhD
Associate Professor
University of Akron
Akron, Ohio

Laralea Stalkie, RN, BNSc, MSN
Professor of Nursing
St. Lawrence College and Laurentian
    University
Kingston, Ontario

D. Shane Strickland, RN, MScN
Lecturer
Lakehead University
Thunder Bay, Ontario

Landa Terblanche, PhD, RN
Associate Professor
Trinity Western University
Langley, British Columbia

Sharon J. Thompson, PhD, RN, MPH
Associate Professor
Gannon University
Erie, Pennsylvania

Patricia Woods, RN, BSN, MSN
Faculty
Langara College
Vancouver, British Columbia

Table of Contents

1

Interpersonal Communication: The Foundation for Patient-Safe Communication

CHAPTER 1

Communication and Patient Safety: Understanding the Connection

Learning Outcomes

Upon completion of this chapter, you will be able to:

Describe the magnitude of communication problems affecting patient safety in health care.

1. Compare sentinel, adverse, and harmful events.
2. Explain the role responsibilities of nurses that involve patient-safe communication.
3. Describe the connection between communication and patient safety.
4. Describe where communication breakdowns occur and how they can lead to harmful events.
5. Identify the key organizations that are addressing communication and patient safety at national and global levels.

Key Terms

Sentinel event
Adverse event
Harmful event

Unshared information
Shared information
Decision-relevant Information

P atient safety always comes first whenever health care is provided. The purpose of this chapter is to describe the fundamental connection between patient safety and communication. Nursing students must develop knowledge and expertise in communication with the same dedication they learn to use a stethoscope and other medical instruments. Patient-safe communication is the key instrument used by nurses and all health-care providers to prevent communication breakdowns and promote patient safety across health-care settings. This chapter introduces the nurse's role responsibilities that involve patient-safe communication. If communication breaks down at any point, patient safety may be compromised and result in serious consequences. Nursing students need to be aware of the latest developments in patient-safe communication strategies.

THE MAGNITUDE OF COMMUNICATION PROBLEMS AND HARMFUL EVENTS

In 1999, the Institute of Medicine (IOM) released a landmark report called, "To Err is Human: Building a Safer Health System."[1] The report estimated that *44,000 to 98,000 people die annually from medical errors in U.S. hospitals.* This means that one patient dies approximately every 5 to 10 minutes in U.S. hospitals. An analysis of over 2000 sentinel events that occurred in health-care organizations in the United States demonstrated that *70% resulted from breakdown in communication.*[2] To view the medical error/sentinel event problem from a different perspective, more people die in a given year as a result of medical errors than from motor vehicle accidents (43,458), breast cancer (42,297), or AIDS (16,516).[3] In Canada, results from a 2004 landmark study revealed that approximately 9000 to 24,000 Canadians die from adverse events in hospitals every year and that more than half of the adverse events were considered preventable.[4]

United States sentinel events and Canadian adverse events are primarily the result of breakdowns in communication. In the U.S. literature, a sentinel event is defined as an unexpected occurrence that results in death or serious physical or psychological injury to a patient. Such an event is called sentinel because it signals the need for immediate investigation.[5] In the Canadian literature, an adverse event is a more general term, defined as an untoward, undesirable, and usually unanticipated patient event, even when there is no permanent effect on the patient.[5] Therefore, sentinel events always involve errors leading to death or permanent disability, whereas adverse events include permanent and potential events leading to death and permanent disability. To avoid confusion over the terms sentinel and adverse events, this book uses the term "harmful event."

The question that needs to be answered at this point is: where does communication break down and cause a harmful event? To answer this question, we introduce the nurse's role responsibilities that involve the crucial need for patient-safe communication and then explain the connection between patient-safe communication and prevention of patient harm.

PATIENT-SAFE COMMUNICATION

Patient-safe communication in nursing is a goal-oriented activity focused on helping patients attain optimal health outcomes. It is the means by which nurses gather and share information, clarify and verify accurate interpretations of information, and establish a process of working collaboratively with patients, their families, and other health-care providers to achieve common goals of safe, high-quality patient care. There are six primary areas of role responsibility of nurses where communication may break down:

1. *Establish the nurse-patient relationship*: to build trust and rapport with the patient. Through trust and rapport, patients are more open to sharing personal health information and to describing how they are feeling and how they are coping with the stress of illness.
2. *Exchange necessary information with the patient:* to keep patients and their families informed; to assess health status, plan interventions, and determine response to treatments and effectiveness of patient teaching.
3. *Ensure accuracy in delivering the correct treatment regime to the correct patient:* to verify patient identification prior to administering any treatment and to actively involve the patient in the process of care whenever possible.
4. *Exchange essential patient information with other health-care providers*: to receive information from and to provide information to members of the health-care team to plan care and to work collaboratively to deliver integrated interdisciplinary care services.
5. *Transfer responsibility of care of the patient and essential patient information to another:* to hand off care and responsibility of the patient to another nurse when leaving the unit for scheduled breaks, to another nursing team during change of shift, or to another nursing unit or health-care agency during patient transfer/discharge.
6. *Ensure accuracy in interpreting information:* to ensure information exchanged between nurses and patients and other members of the health-care team is interpreted as intended.

The consequences of communication breakdowns during performance of these role responsibilities jeopardizes patient safety. Next, we examine the direct connection between communication and patient safety.

CONNECTION BETWEEN COMMUNICATION AND PATIENT SAFETY

The critical connection between communication and patient safety is that nurses and other health-care providers *make clinical decisions, plan treatments, and perform interventions on patients based on available information that is communicated between health-care team members and patients.* It is important to understand that every aspect of patient care hinges on how health-care team members, including patients, have interpreted available information. If clinical decisions are based on incomplete or misinterpreted information, treatments may be planned and performed by health-care providers that are inappropriate and may cause patient harm.

Making Clinical Decisions Based on Patient Sharing of Personal Health Information

To promote patient safety, nurses and other health-care providers must communicate with patients in a way that encourages the patients to share personal health information. This is accomplished by building trust, which is the foundation of the provider-patient relationship. Nurses and other health-care providers use specific patient-safe communication strategies to develop, nurture, and maintain the trusting relationship. If patients do not feel a sense of trust in and genuine sincerity from those involved in their care, they may not share information that is necessary for accurate decision making and treatment planning. As an example, if the nurse appears rushed or distracted while she is conducting the patient's health history, the patient may abbreviate his responses. He may not mention that he has allergies to certain medications, for instance. Without this essential information, the patient may be prescribed a medication that can cause a harmful allergic reaction, which becomes a sentinel event.

Nurses and other health-care providers ensure that they have accurately identified the patient when gathering health information and prior to administering treatments. Through this critical communication behavior, nurses can avoid administering the wrong treatments to patients.

Making Clinical Decisions Based on Sharing Patient Information

The most appropriate and safe patient care requires effective sharing of information among members of the health-care team.[7] Essential patient information known by an individual health-care provider must be communicated or shared with other professionals involved in the patient's care.[8,9] The theory linking sharing of patient information and patient safety is supported by the information-pooling model of communication proposed by Stasser and Titus.[10,11] Their model suggests that group members who have diverse stores of information as a result of differences in training, experience, and role may often hold a certain amount of decision-relevant information that other members of the group do not have. This uniquely held knowledge by one member of the group is called unshared information. Unshared information may be critical to the overall quality of the group's decision making. By pooling unshared information, groups have the potential for making more informed decisions than if decisions were made on uniquely held information of any individual.

When applying this model to health care, it stands to reason that each team member from different disciplines may hold unique information about the patient because of his specific role and area of expertise. When disciplines share their information, there is greater access to information for decision making by the entire interdisciplinary health-care team.

If essential patient information is not shared, this leads to gaps in communication that can create serious breakdowns in the continuity of care, lead to inappropriate treatment, and ultimately harm patients.[12] A gap is a breakdown in communication. For example, if a patient tells the nurse that his breathing is becoming more difficult and the nurse does not share this information, the amount of information accessible for decision making by the physician and other members of the health-care team decreases, thereby increasing the potential for patient harm. Likewise, if there are delays in receiving information from laboratory results or x-ray reports, team members that make clinical decisions in the absence of this information may do so in error.

Ensuring Accuracy: Conveying and Interpreting Messages Accurately

As important as it is to share essential information to promote appropriate decision making and patient safety, it is equally important to ensure that the information is conveyed and interpreted *accurately*. Accuracy in shared patient information is always dependent on the communication skill of the individual.[13,14] For example, nurses must communicate effectively using clear and concise language to ensure that verbal messages containing essential patient information are conveyed to members of the health-care team as accurately as possible. This increases the ability of others to interpret patient information as intended. Statements from one nurse to another such as, "He is a bit nauseated" or "My patients are all OK, I am going to take my break" are vague, ambiguous, open to misinterpretation, and do not provide adequate information for others to make accurate clinical decisions.[15,16] Misinterpretations are breakdowns in communication that can lead to errors in decision making and inappropriate treatment planning that may result in a harmful event.

Knowing that even the most clear and precise verbal message can be misinterpreted, nurses must always seek feedback to determine how another team member has interpreted their messages. Through this communication behavior, nurses can offer clarification if needed and confirm accuracy of interpretation to ensure that patient information has been understood fully by others. Through this same process, nurses ensure that they have interpreted the information they receive from other health-care providers as intended.

When communicating with patients, nurses must understand that many factors can interfere with the patient's ability to convey and interpret messages accurately. As examples, factors may include pain, anxiety, health literacy, and sensory impairments. Nurses must use clear language that is appropriate to the age and stage of development of the patient to overcome any factors that may interfere with the patient's ability to interpret messages accurately. When nurses convey information to patients, they seek feedback from them to ensure that patients have interpreted their messages accurately. Professionally educated in patient-safe communication, nurses and other health-care providers bear the greater responsibility of ensuring accuracy in communication during their interactions and information exchange with patients.

When patients share personal health information with nurses, nurses must proceed with high-level communication competency to provide appropriate feedback to patients to confirm that they have accurately interpreted patients' messages as intended.

 INITIATIVES TO IMPROVE COMMUNICATION AND PATIENT SAFETY

Initiatives to reduce the risk of harmful events caused by problems with communication have become a national and global focus, led by such organizations as the U.S. Joint Commission, the Canadian Council on Health Services Accreditation, and the World Health Organization.

The Joint Commission and the Canadian Council on Health Services Accreditation

The role of the Joint Commission and the Canadian Council on Health Services Accreditation is to examine and improve the quality of care and services provided to patients by health-care organizations.[17,18] These organizations set the standards of quality care and measure hospitals and other health-care organizations' compliance with these standards. The Joint Commission and the Canadian Council have developed national patient safety goals for improving communication among health-care providers.[19,20] To support achievement of these goals is a series of standards in communication. Hospitals and other health-care organizations, too, are designing patient-safe communication strategies to meet these standards and improve patient safety and reduce the potential for harmful events.

World Health Organization

In 2004, the World Health Organization (WHO) launched the World Alliance for Patient Safety.[21] The Alliance coordinates, disseminates, and accelerates improvements in patient safety worldwide, highlighting safety as a global issue for patients in countries rich and poor, developed and developing. The WHO Collaborating Center for Patient Safety was established in 2005 and focuses worldwide attention on patient safety solutions that can reduce patient harm and coordinates international efforts to spread these solutions as broadly as possible.[22] The WHO Collaborating Center has developed several patient safety solutions specific to improving communication in health care. The WHO defines patient safety solutions as "any system design or intervention that has demonstrated the ability to prevent or mitigate patient harm stemming from the processes of health care."[12]

Many patient safety communication concepts and specific communication strategies introduced in this book stem from the recommendations of the Joint Commission, the Canadian Patient Safety Institute and the Canadian Council on Health Services Accreditation, and from the WHO. Collectively, the communication concepts and strategies used in patient care will be referred to as patient-safe communication strategies within this book.

Evidence-Based Research

Health-care professionals recognize the substantial improvements to quality in patient care that result from implementing evidence-based research into clinical practice. Within the nursing profession, clinical practice that is evidence-based provides a strong scientific foundation for nursing practice.[23] The use of patient-safe communication strategies to decrease patient injury and death has not been researched with the rigorous testing required meeting evidence-based research standards. Research studies are, however, currently under way.

One key concern, however, for health-care organizations and professionals is that it takes approximately 10 to 17 years for research findings to be translated fully into practice.[24] Patients, health-care providers, and the health-care system cannot wait that long. There is great opportunity now to integrate patient-safe practices in communication developed by leading patient safety organizations, which have been endorsed worldwide by safety experts, nursing and medical profession associations, and health-care organizations. "No adverse event should ever occur anywhere in the world if the knowledge exists to prevent it from happening."[25]

CHAPTER SUMMARY

Communication is the key instrument for patient safety used by nurses and all health-care providers to ensure the ongoing accuracy and continuity of patient information to promote safe, quality care. Gaps in communication and misinterpretations pose risks to patient safety and can result in patient harm. It is critical that nurses develop high-level competence in communication and use patient-safe communication strategies provided by the leading experts nationally and worldwide to keep patients safe from harm and to build a safer health-care system.

BUILDING HIGH LEVEL COMMUNICATION COMPETENCE

For additional exercises, visit DavisPlus at http://davisplus.fadavis.com

1. **Reflection.** Think about a time you misinterpreted communication. Think about how easy and common it is to misinterpret messages. Think also of times when you have said, "Well, had I known that, I would have...." This is a classic example of gaps in communication.

2. **Critical Thinking Exercise.** How can this nurse's statement to the oncoming nurse as she hands off care and responsibility lead to a harmful event: "My patients are all OK—I am off for break."

References

1. Institute of Medicine: To Err is Human: Building a Safer Health System. A Report of the Committee on Quality of Health Care in America. National Academy Press, 1999. www.iom.edu/Object.File/Master/4/117/ToErr-8pager.pdf Accessed December 2008.
2. Joint Commission, 2004: Sentinel Event Statistics, June 29, 2004, as cited in Leonard, M., Graham, S., Bonacum, D. The Human Factor: The Critical Importance of Effective Teamwork and Communication in Providing Safe Care. Quality and Safety in Health Care 13:i85-i90, 2004.
3. Centers for Disease Control and Prevention (National Center for Health Statistics). Births and Deaths: Preliminary Data for 1998. National Vital Statistic Reports 47:6, 1999.
4. Baker, C., Norton, P., Flintoft, V., et al. The Canadian Adverse Events Study: The Incidence of Adverse Events Among Hospital Patients in Canada. CMAJ 170:1678-1686, 2004.
5. Joint Commission, 2008. FAQs for the 2008 National Patient Safety Goals. www.jointcommission.org/NR/rdonlyres/13234515-DD9A-4635-A718-D5E84A98AF13/0/2008_FAQs_NPSG_02.pdf Accessed January 2009.
6. Kohn, L.T., Corrigan, J.M., Donaldson, M.S. (eds.). To Err is Human: Building a Safer Health System. Washington, DC, National Academy Press, Institute of Medicine: 2000.
7. Spath, P. Reducing Errors Through Work System Improvements. In Spath, P. (ed.). Error Reduction in Health Care, 199-234. San Francisco, Jossey-Bass: 2000.
8. Institute of Medicine: Crossing the Quality Chasm: A New Health System for the 21st Century. Washington, DC, Committee on the Quality Health Care in America, National Academy of Sciences, National Academy Press: 2001.
9. Anthony, M.K. Models of Care: The Influence of Nurse Communication on Patient Safety. Nursing Economics. findarticles.com/p/articles/mi_m0FSW/is_5_20/ai_n18614298 Accessed May 2008.
10. Stasser, G., Titus, W. Pooling of Unshared Information in Group Decision Making: Biased Information Sampling During Discussion. Journal of Personality and Social Psychology 48:1467-1478, 1985.
11. Stasser, G., Titus, W. Effects of Information Load and Percentage of Shared Information on the Dissemination of Unshared Information During Group Discussion. Journal of Personality and Social Psychology 53:81-93, 1987.
12. World Health Organization, 2007. Communications During Patient Handovers: Patient Safety Solutions. http://www.jcipatientsafety.org/fpdf/presskit/PS- Solution3.pdf Accessed May 2008.
13. Friesen, M.A., White, S.V., Byers, J.F. Hand-Offs: Implications for Nurses. In Hughes, R.G. (ed.). Patient Safety and Quality: An Evidence-Based Handbook for Nurses Agency for Healthcare Research and Quality. Publication No. 08-0043., Rockville, Md. www.ahrq.gov/qual/nurseshdbk Accessed January 2008.
14. Australian Council for Safety and Quality in Health Care 2005. Clinical Handover and Patient Safety Literature Review Report: Safety and Quality Council. www.safetyandquality.org Accessed May 2008.
15. Joint Commission. Focus on Five: Strategies to Improve Hand-Off Communications: Implementing a Process to Resolve Questions. Joint Commission Perspectives on Patient Safety 5:11, 2005.
16. Evanoff, B., Potter, P., Wolf, L., et al. Can We Talk? Priorities for Patient Care Differed Among Health Providers. In Henriksen, K., Battles, J.B., Marks, E., et al. (eds.). Advances in Patient Safety: From Research to Implementation, vol 1, Research Findings. Rockville, Md: Agency for Healthcare Research and Quality Publication No. 05-0021-1, 2005.

17. The Joint Commission. About Us. www.jointcommission.org/AboutUs/joint_commission_facts.htm Accessed October 2007.
18. Canadian Patient Safety Institute. About Us. www.patientsafetyinstitute.ca/about.html Accessed November 2007.
19. The Joint Commission. National Patient Safety Goals, 2009. www.jointcommission.org/GeneralPublic/NPSG/09_npsgs.htm
20. Organizational Practices (ROPs): New ROPs for 2009 Accreditation Surveys. www.accreditation-canada.ca Accessed November 2008.
21. World Health Organization, 2004. About Us. www.who.int/patientsafety/about/en/index.html Accessed September 2008.
22. World Health Organization, 2005. News Release: World Health Organization Partners With Joint Commission and Joint Commission International to Eliminate Errors Worldwide. Oakbrook Terrace, Ill. www.who.int/patientsafety/newsalert/WHO_final.pdf Accessed November 2008.
23. Timmermans, S., Mauck, A. The Promises and Pitfalls of Evidence-Based Medicine. Health Affairs 24:18-28, 2005.
24. Balas, A.E., Borem, S.A. Managing Clinical Knowledge for Health Care Improvement. Yearbook of Medical Informatics. Bethesda, Md., National Library of Medicine: 2000, 65-71.
25. World Health Organization, 2009. Patient Safety Solutions. www.who.int/patientsafety/solutions/patientsafety/en/ Accessed March 2009.

The Patient-Safe Transformational Model of Communication

Learning Outcomes

Upon completion of this chapter, you will be able to:

1. Define high-level communication competence.
2. Describe the effects of interpersonal communication on relationships.
3. Explain the evolution of communication models.
4. Describe the elements of the transformational model of communication.
5. Define communication using the transformational model of communication.
6. Identify the principles of communication.

Key Terms

Communicators
Critical thought processing
Message
Channel
Assign meaning
Effects

Feedback
Validation
Context
Communication risk factors
Patient-safe communication strategies
Transformation

ow that you are aware of the connection between communication and patient safety, this chapter will introduce you to the basic concepts of communication. You will begin by assessing your current level of competency in communication. Because communication is central to human existence and the means by which people form and manage relationships, this chapter focuses on interpersonal communication and relationships as the foundation upon which professional nurse-patient and interdisciplinary team communication and relationships are built. The chapter describes how understanding of communication has evolved over time and led to the development of the transformational model of communication. The transformational model is a framework for communicating with high-level competence. It has been used to organize the content of this book and to help you gain the foundational knowledge needed to become a patient-safe communicator.

HOW WELL DO YOU COMMUNICATE?

Communication is central to our lives. Nevertheless, we rarely give it any thought until we have had either a bad experience, such as a disagreement that turned nasty, or an exhilarating experience like having a good interview and getting the job. Every day, we experience communication more than any other human activity.

Communication is a complex process. What we say and how we say it are influenced by who we are and how we perceive the world. Sometimes we must work very hard to understand the thoughts and feelings that are unique to the person with whom we communicate. Establishing a common understanding between people is the challenge in communication and is critical to patient safety. For an interactive version of this activity, visit DavisPlus at http://davisplus.fadavis.com

HIGH-LEVEL COMMUNICATION COMPETENCY

Learning to communicate with high-level competency is the main reason to study communication. Although the term competency holds a variety of meanings, it is generally defined as a cluster of related knowledge, skills, and attitudes or motivation that individuals need to possess to perform their role or a particular task.[1,2] In terms of communication competence, knowledge means knowing what behavior is best suited for a given situation. Skill is having the ability to apply the behavior in the given context. Attitude or motivation is having the desire to communicate in a competent manner.[1] High-level communication competence can then be defined by the following knowledge, skills, and attitude:

1. The ability to choose communication behaviors that are effective and appropriate for a given situation[3]
2. The ability to be sensitive to the perspectives of others, and
3. The ability to achieve communication goals in a manner that maintains or enhances the relationship in which it occurs.[4]

Effective communication occurs when messages are understood by others as intended.[3] Individuals with high-level competency accomplish this by choosing communication behaviors that convey messages clearly and precisely, leaving interpretation less open to chance. High-level communicators must also choose communication behaviors to help ensure they understand the messages of others as the others intend. High-level communicators accomplish this by offering and seeking clarifications to ensure a high probability that messages are interpreted as intended.

Appropriateness in communication occurs when people assess the context of a situation and adapt communication accordingly.[3] We speak differently when communicating with a toddler, a police officer, and a good friend. *Sensitivity* in communication entails recognizing the feelings and perspectives of others that differ from our own.[4] It allows us to hear the perspectives of others without judgment and to accept the uniqueness of each person.

Achieving communication goals in a manner that maintains the relationship is called *saving face.* Saving face means making choices on how you respond to others, maintaining respect for others and for yourself, and managing the impressions of yourself you wish to project.[4] Figure 2.1 illustrates the four components that define high-level communication competency.

People who have not developed high-level competence in communication are limited in their efforts to achieve personal and professional goals. For both professional and interpersonal relationships you need to know how to speak clearly, listen effectively, clarify interpretations, be empathetic, deal with conflict, and understand communication styles that differ from your own. In professional relationships with patients, these communication competencies provide the foundation for developing trust, encouraging patient sharing of health information, helping patients cope with illness, and providing health education ensuring that patients interpret and understand the information correctly and as intended. In professional relationships with other health-care providers, these competencies are the foundation for sharing patient information accurately for appropriate clinical decision making and for working with other disciplines to provide safe, quality care.

CONCEPTS OF INTERPERSONAL COMMUNICATION AND INTERPERSONAL RELATIONSHIPS

Humans are social beings. We derive satisfaction from interacting with others, and we use communication as a means to initiate these opportunities. *Interpersonal communication* is a form of communication that is used when we view others as unique individuals and interact with them for the purpose of maintaining an ongoing relationship.[5] Interpersonal communications are open, honest, nonjudgmental, and based on equality (Buber, 1958).[6] Interpersonal communication allows us to gain knowledge about others so we can interact

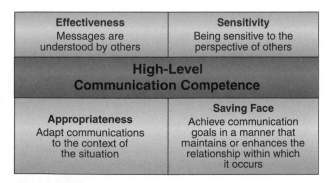

Effectiveness	Sensitivity
Messages are understood by others	Being sensitive to the perspective of others
High-Level Communication Competence	
Appropriateness Adapt communications to the context of the situation	**Saving Face** Achieve communication goals in a manner that maintains or enhances the relationship within which it occurs

Figure 2.1 Concepts of high-level communication competence.

with them more easily. By knowing others better, we are more able to predict how they will respond to us, and we can adapt our communications accordingly.

An *interpersonal relationship* is the enduring connection that we make with others through interpersonal communication.[7] The interpersonal relationship is characterized by trust and honesty in sharing thoughts and feelings within a context of genuine acceptance of the differences between individuals. We develop our sense of belonging, worth, and acceptance through interpersonal relationships.

EVOLUTION OF MODELS OF COMMUNICATION

Communication has its theoretical roots in the fields of telecommunication and psychotherapy.[8,9] Although our understanding of the communication process has evolved over the past 60 years, basic definitions remain unchanged from the original models. They are the linear, interactional, and transactional models of the communication process.

Message Transmission: The Linear Model

In the late 1940s Claude Shannon, an applied mathematician and engineer who worked for Bell Telephone Laboratories, was charged with ensuring the maximum efficiency of telephone cables and radio waves. He developed a model that reduced the communication process to a set of seven basic elements: sender, receiver, encode, decode, message, channel, and noise.[8] He, along with other scholars of that era, described the first notions of how communication happened and why it sometimes failed.[10]

These early models depicted communication as a linear, one-way process where messages were transmitted in a straightforward manner from one person to another. See Figure 2.2, which illustrates a linear model of communication.

In simple terms, a *sender* was the originator of a message who *encoded* or determined what and how to say the message. The sender transmitted the *message* through a particular *channel,* such as a phone or in person, to a *receiver* who would interpret or *decode* the message. Communication could fail because of *noise,* which included any distortion that could interfere with the integrity or accuracy of the message, such as static on a phone line or talking inaudibly.

Message Exchange: The Interactional Model

As scholars continued to study communication, they realized that human conversation was much more than a one-way process. In 1954 Wilbur Schramm developed the interactional

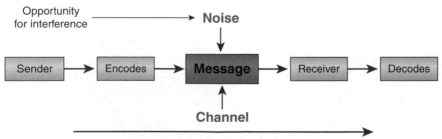

Sender sends a message; receiver receives message passively

Figure 2.2 Linear model of communication.

model of communication.[11] The model introduced the element of *feedback* to reflect the two-way flow of communication between people. See Figure 2.3, which illustrates the interactional model of communication. In addition, this model also introduced the element of *fields of experience*. As Foulger[10] indicated, this acknowledged that people create and interpret messages within their own unique perspectives, experiences, culture, and history.

Shared Message Creation: The Transactional Model

Scholars such as Barnlund[12] developed the transactional model of communication in 1970. The transactional model described the communication process as a reciprocal, simultaneous flow of messages and feedback between individuals as shown in Figure 2.4. The model illustrated that while people speak, they are busy interpreting their partner's nonverbal and verbal responses. Senders and receivers were redefined as *communicators* to reflect the simultaneous flow of messages and feedback during conversations.

In the transactional model, communication was described as a process of negotiating and creating common meaning. Encoding and decoding were mutually interdependent actions of the communicators, each contributing to the shared meaning they were building together.[13] The element of *context* was introduced, which expanded the original element of fields of experience in the interactional model. Through awareness of context, communicators acknowledged factors, such as the physical and social setting, time of communication, and the emotions and mood of the communicators, that could influence the communication situation. The transactional model acknowledged that creation and interpretation of messages evolves from the past, is influenced by the present, and is affected by visions of the future.[7]

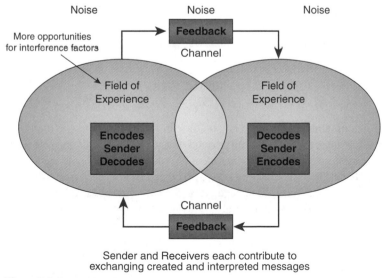

Sender and Receivers each contribute to
exchanging created and interpreted messages

Figure 2.3 Interactional model of communication.

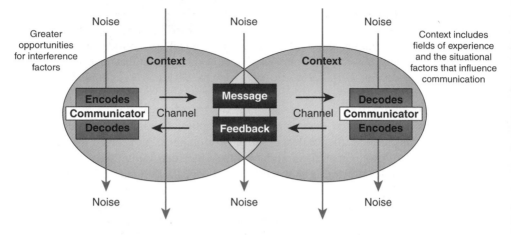

Communicators create and send messages simultaneously
and are equally responsible for creating common meaning

Figure 2.4 Transactional model of communication.

In this same era, the element of noise evolved to include:

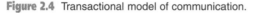

- Psychological noise: the emotional state of the communicators, their personalities and preconceived ideas and judgments.
- Physical noise: external factors that distract communicators like loud music in the background or being unfamiliar with the physical setting.
- Physiological noise: the biological factors that interfere with communications such as fatigue, illness, or altered cognitive function.
- Semantic noise: the way people speak, their use of terms, and any dialect or literacy issues.

This book introduces the transformational model of communication to be used as a practical guide for interpersonal communication and professional patient-safe communication. In the transformational model, the focus is on the effects of messages and achieving desired outcomes.

✦ CREATING EFFECTS AND OUTCOMES: A TRANSFORMATIONAL MODEL OF COMMUNICATION

Whenever we communicate, we have an outcome in mind. The outcome might be as simple as enjoying a relaxing conversation with a friend or as complex as calming down a highly anxious patient to administer a prescribed treatment. Whether we achieve our desired outcome depends on the effects our communications have on others. Effective messages are conveyed and interpreted as intended. Effects are dependent on the appropriateness of our communications, how sensitive we are to others, and our ability to save face for self and others.

The transformational model is focused on high-level competency to create specific effects to achieve desired communication outcomes. Communication breakdown is the major contributor to harmful events, including injury and death, in health-care settings. Harmful events are undesired outcomes. Whether a patient had the wrong limb amputated or suffered renal damage as a result of errors in clinical decision making that were caused by communication breakdowns, the nature, form, appearance, character, or condition of the individual was changed.

In contrast to the negative outcomes of communication, there are examples of positive transformations that happen every day. Education is a classic example of the transformational process of communication. The outcome of education is, for example, transforming a lay person into a professional nurse. The values, attitudes, and knowledge that are required have been communicated through written, verbal, and nonverbal communication from faculty, peers, and preceptors. Figure 2.5 illustrates the transformational model of communication. The model consists of 12 interacting elements of the communication process within a central core and surrounding rings.

Within the central core are two unique individuals communicating. They are sharing information, providing each other with feedback to create a common understanding of each other's messages, and creating specific effects to achieve specific desired outcomes through communication. Communicators are influenced by the context of the communication situation (first ring) and communication risk factors inherent within the communication situation (second ring). Communicators can use patient-safe communication strategies to overcome

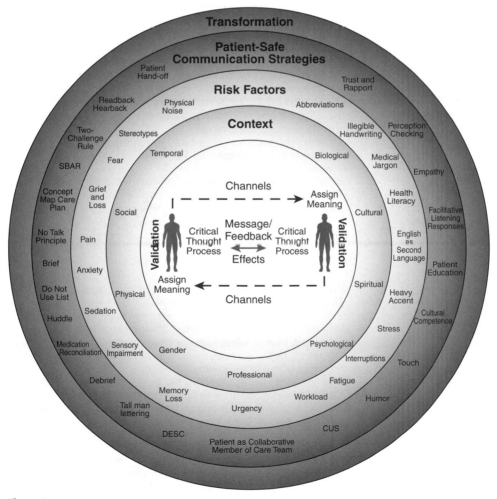

Figure 2.5 Transformational model of communication.

risk factors (third ring). In the outer ring is the transformational outcome of the communication process. A summary of definitions of the elements of the communication process within the transformational model appears in Table 2.1.

A description of each of the twelve elements begins at the core of the model.

TABLE 2.1 Definitions of Elements of the Communication Process

Element	Description
(1) Communicators	Originators of facts, thoughts, or feelings Unique bio-psycho-social-cultural-spiritual beings Each communicates to meet human needs; includes physical, social, identity, and practical needs Each is transformed by the communications
(2) Critical thought processing	Cognitive deliberations used during communication to: • Determine the human need that must be met and the desired communication outcome • Assess the communication situation including the individual, environment, and actual/potential risk factors • Select communication strategies to overcome risk factors • Create the message by means of effective, appropriate, sensitive, and face-saving verbal and nonverbal behaviors • Choose the best channel for conveying the message • Evaluate the effects and responses of messages and adjust communications accordingly • Facilitate common meaning through feedback to ensure messages are interpreted as intended
(3) Message	Contains the facts, thoughts, or feelings of a communicator that are conveyed to another through words and nonverbal clues that enable individuals to assign meaning to the message Includes content and relational dimensions May be intentional or unintentional; are unrepeatable and irreversible Verbal behavior includes spoken, written, or electronic words Nonverbal behavior includes gestures, eye contact, body language, and tone of voice
(4) Channel	Method or pathway by which the message is conveyed; for example, face to face, letters, e-mail, Internet, phone call, or mass media, such as newspaper, television, radio, movies
(5) Assign meaning	Communicators assign meaning to the message based on their individual uniqueness, life experiences, context, content, relational dimensions of messages, and how well communicators know one another
(6) Effects	All messages cause reactions in communicators, which may be the desired effect or an unanticipated effect Effects influence outcomes of the communication situation May be intentional or unintentional; are unrepeatable and irreversible

TABLE 2.1 (continued)	
Element	**Description**
(7) Feedback	Verbal and nonverbal response to a message
(8) Validation	Validation is an attempt to create common meaning Communicators clarify and verify through feedback that the intended meaning of the message has been correctly interpreted
(9) Communicators in context	The tangible and intangible environment in which communication occurs and influences the communication situation Includes physical, temporal, social, biological, gender, psychological, cultural, spiritual, and professional contexts
(10) Communication risk factors	Anything that potentially or actually interferes with clear communication Includes physical, psychological, physiological, and semantic risk factors
(11) Patient-safe communication strategies	Structured, purposeful communication strategies used to overcome communication risk factors when interacting professionally with patients, interdisciplinary health professionals, and during specific error-prone moments within the health-care continuum
(12) Transformation	An outcome of the communication process Includes affective, cognitive, psychomotor, and bio-psycho-social-spiritual cultural changes in people as a result of the communication experience

Element No. 1: Communicators

Each communicator is a unique bio-psycho-social-cultural-spiritual being. At least two people communicate to meet human needs; therefore, communication is goal-oriented. Communicators are the originators of facts, thoughts, or feelings that are expressed to meet physical, social, identity, and practical needs.

Physical Needs

Humans communicate to meet physical needs. Communication is so important to our lives that, without it, we can become physically ill. The research linking physical illness with lack of meaningful human interaction has received international attention through the World Health Organization (WHO). The WHO published a report[14] summarizing the social determinants of health and concluded that social isolation increased rates of premature death and lowered chances of survival after a heart attack. Additionally, the report suggested that individuals lacking interaction are more likely to experience less well-being, more depression, a greater risk of pregnancy complications, and higher levels of disability from chronic disease.

Social Needs

In addition to promoting health and well being, communication provides a vital connection to others. Researchers have identified many social needs that are satisfied by communicating with others, including the need to share a story, have fun, be consoled, express emotions, gain another's perspective, and feel connected to others.[15] Through social interactions with others, we also learn what is and is not acceptable behavior and how to adjust our behavior to maintain social expectations at home, work, and with friends. We learn social interaction skills through communicating with others who give us cues on how to relate within different social situations. It is through these experiences that we learn about appropriateness of communication.

Identity Needs

Communication enables us to learn who we are.[16] Our sense of identity comes mainly from our interactions with others and our perception of their responses to us. Do their responses tell us we have a good sense of humor, or do they say we are too serious? Do they let us know that we are warm and friendly, or do they give us the sense that we are confrontational and insincere? Deprived of communication with others, we would have little way of knowing the person we are.

Practical Needs

We would not be able to survive if we did not communicate our practical needs. We tell a server what we want to order for lunch or describe to a clerk the type of coat we want to buy. We may need to learn a new role, understand the tasks associated with a new job, or how to coach and teach others. In health-care settings, patients have a practical need to let their caregivers know their health concerns. They also have the practical need to ask questions about their health status, treatments, and medications and how to manage self-care when they are discharged home.

Communication Safety Alert

Nurses must assess which human needs patients may express directly or indirectly. Patients will never say, "I have a need for social connectedness." Nurses can, however, be alert for vulnerable populations such as women and the elderly where research has shown the effects of lack of social support on their health.

Element No. 2: Critical Thought Processing

Critical thought processing reflects the cognitive deliberations used by communicators in their attempt to achieve common understanding, specific effects, and desired outcomes. The purpose of critical thought processing is to:

- Determine the human need that must be met and the desired communication outcome
- Assess the communication situation (communicators, context, risk factors)
- Select communication strategies to overcome risk factors
- Create the message by choosing effective, appropriate, sensitive, and face-saving verbal and nonverbal behaviors
- Choose the best channel for conveying the message
- Evaluate the effects and responses of messages and adjust communications accordingly
- Facilitate common meaning so that messages are interpreted as intended

Element No. 3: Message

Messages contain the facts, thoughts, or feelings of a communicator that are conveyed to another through verbal and nonverbal behavior. Verbal behavior refers to spoken, written, or electronic words. Words are open to interpretation, and it is likely that no two people will interpret the same word in exactly the same way. This is because words themselves do not have meaning; rather, meaning resides in the people who express and interpret them.[17] Consider, for example, the word "exciting." What mental image immediately came to mind? What associations did you attach to this word? Undoubtedly, you would not find another person with the exact image and associations you had. The reason for these differences is that the word exciting contains no meaning. Meaning comes from individuals and is influenced by their unique perspectives. This explains why it is necessary for communicators to try to convey, as accurately as possible, the intended meaning of a message and highlights the importance of effectiveness in communication. Individuals, all of whom have a life history different from yours, may have difficulty interpreting your message as intended. If you are vague, messages may be misinterpreted. This can happen even with people who know you well, such as people in your family. How communication is influenced by our unique perspectives is discussed in Chapter 3, in which perceptions and sense of self are discussed. Ways to create and interpret messages accurately are examined in Chapter 4.

Nonverbal behavior refers to behaviors such as gestures, facial expressions, and tone of voice. Nonverbal behavior illustrates how we cannot avoid communicating. For example, if you attempt not to communicate by avoiding eye contact or deliberately remaining silent, you are still communicating messages to others. *All observed behavior has communicative value.*

In contrast to conveying deliberate nonverbal behaviors, most often our nonverbal behavior happens unconsciously and escapes our ability to apply critical thought processing. This makes it difficult to plan which types of nonverbal behaviors we will choose to use in our message. Through verbal communications with others, we gain insight into our nonverbal behaviors that escaped concious thought.

Messages contain both a content and a relational dimension. Content refers to *what* is said through verbal behavior such as facts, opinions, and thoughts. Relational refers to *how* it was said, the tone of the voice and the nonverbal behavior of body language. The relational dimension offers clues on how communicators feel about each other, their status in the relationship and the amount of power each feels toward the other, and helps others understand the meaning behind the words that are conveyed.[18] The content combined with relational dimensions of the message reveals the true meaning of the message. The relational dimension provides the necessary clues for interpreting the words conveyed in the message.

Element No. 4: Channel

Channel refers to the method or pathway by which messages are communicated. The method we are most familiar with is face-to-face. Face-to-face communication is synchronous, meaning it happens in real life in real time. Verbal and nonverbal messages occur simultaneously, providing a rich flow of immediate feedback for each communicator.

The telephone is a channel that is also in real time. The difference between it and face-to-face is that it does not allow for communicators to see the nonverbal behaviors that accompany the message; they can only hear them through the speaker's voice. Changes in technology have increased our options for conveying messages. Computer-mediated communication (CMC) provides opportunities to communicate messages electronically over the Internet, including e-mail and instant messaging. CMC has advantages and disadvantages. For example, although instant messaging can be considered real-time or synchronous communication, its disadvantage is that communicators are not able to see or hear each other's nonverbal behavior.

Communicators have to rely on emoticons, which are symbols that express emotions and nonverbal gestures in CMC. Some symbols provide clues as to the communication process itself, such as indicating you have just said the wrong thing, made a mistake, or relayed a message that is incoherent. Although the development of additional symbols continues, they cannot fully replace the richness of visual and audible clues we experience in face-to-face conversations.

E-mail has similar limitations as instant messaging, with a variant feature of being asynchronous, or not in real time. Communicators who send messages must wait until a response is e-mailed back to receive feedback, much like the communication process described in the interactional model of communication. Much of the spontaneity and immediate feedback that comes from synchronous communication is diminished in e-mail communications.

There are, however, some clear advantages to consider with e-mail. E-mail can make communications easier in a very busy schedule. Communicators control the time they choose to reply to messages, although as noted previously, this convenience for one communicator can cause frustrations for another. Another advantage of e-mail is that you can rewrite the message until you have expressed exactly what you want, which is not always possible in face-to-face or phone communication. Interpersonal relationships over multiple time zones and long distances can be more easily maintained through CMC where face-to-face conversation may be impossible. Additionally, many new relationships have been initiated via e-mail through Internet dating services and may eventually develop into interpersonal face-to-face relationships.

Other channels of communication include written forms, such as letters, greeting cards, and memos. Like the telephone and CMC, written messages lack the nonverbal component, and feedback response times vary. In health care, there are a variety of specific written channels of communication. They include prescription pads, doctors' order sheets, nursing notes, and vital sign records. The entire patient's health record is a channel for sharing patient information across disciplines, care units, and nursing shifts. Health-care professionals rely on the documentation in the record to provide continuity and safety in patient care. Written communication in health care is discussed in greater detail in Unit 3.

The last channel of communication to address is mass media. Mass media include newspapers, tabloids, journals, books, billboards, radio, movies, and television. Mass media provide one-way communication in that a message is conveyed to many people by a communicator, reflecting the one-way communication process in the linear model of communication. Feedback may only come indirectly by way of television ratings, trends in sales, complaints to the customer service department, or a lawsuit.

Element No. 5: Assign Meaning

Individuals interpret messages based on the meaning they have assigned to the verbal and nonverbal behavior of the communicator. The meaning that is assigned depends on many interacting factors. These factors include the unique perspectives of the communicators, the context of the communication situation, the content and relational dimensions of the message, and any risk factors that may interfere with interpreting the intended meaning of the message accurately. Risk factors can include each communicator's physical and cognitive ability to speak, listen, and interpret messages.

Element No. 6: Effects

Once interpreted, all messages create effects.[17] Effects are a means to an end: the desired outcome of the communication situation. The effect may be happiness, excitement, concern, or fear; interest in the subject being discussed, or disinterest that may shut down communication. The effects of messages are conveyed through verbal and nonverbal feedback.

We are motivated to create a specific effect in another person to achieve a desired communication outcome. We gauge the effects of our messages carefully to determine if they are as intended or if they are unintended. It is important to recognize that effects always happen. For example, even if a message appears to be ignored, the effect is that the communicators felt the message was not important to even address.

The messages and effects created may be intentional or unintentional. You carefully consider your words when you are being interviewed for your first nursing position in order to create a positive effect. Conversely, you might find yourself singing along to a song in your car and notice that you are being observed by the driver in the next lane. You were not intending to communicate a message to an onlooker, but it happened, and you created an unintentional effect.

Element No. 7: Feedback

Feedback is the verbal and nonverbal response to messages that communicators convey to each other. Feedback conveys responses such as the effect of a message, thoughts on the content of the message, feelings associated with the message, interpretation of the message, and the relational aspect of the people and relationships involved in the communication situation. Feedback provides a circular mechanism in communication processes where clarification of interpretations and validation of the meaning of the message can occur. Misinterpretations can be corrected through feedback.

Element No. 8: Validation

Validation is the means by which feedback helps communicators create common meaning. People involved in the communication situation mutually determine whether the messages are understood, if there is need for clarification, or if the message must be completely restated in order to be fully understood. Communicators clarify and verify that the interpretation of the message by the receiver matches the intended meaning of the sender. Through clarifying and verifying messages, common meaning may be negotiated and mutually agreed upon by the communicators.

It is important to understand that validation applies to both the verbal and nonverbal aspects of a message. Think of times you have been preoccupied with another matter while communicating with someone. The preoccupation can come across in your tone or facial expression as boredom with the current discussion. When the individual you were speaking with calls attention to your behavior, you can clarify the situation and avoid misinterpretations and a communciation breakdown. Through validating both verbal and nonverbal aspects of messages, communicators are prevented from making interpretation errors during communication.

Element No. 9: Communicators in Context

All communication takes place within a contex.[17] Context refers to the tangible and intangible environment in which communication occurs and influences the communication situation. There are physical, temporal, gender, biological, cultural, psychological, social, spiritual, and professional contexts in this ring. In any communication situation, several contexts may be interacting at the same time.

The *physical* context provides the tangible structure where messages are shared and influences the appropriateness of communication choices. As examples, the physical context may be a home, classroom, office, church, or hospital.

The *temporal* context refers to the timing of communication. This includes day, week, season, or significant event in a person's history.

The *gender* context refers to differences in how men and women communicate and the influence of these differences during conversations. Gender differences in communication are the focus of Chapter 5.

The *biological* context takes into consideration the appearance and level of functioning of the communicators. For example, we adjust our communication when we interact with individuals in a wheelchair to deliver a message effectively. We will sit or bend to talk with them at the same eye level.

The *cultural* context refers to the norms, traditions, and customs that affect interpersonal communication. In some cultures, it is impolite to establish direct eye contact; there may be rules that dictate who speaks first. Cultural competence is discussed in Chapter 5.

The *psychological* context refers to the aspects of emotion, mood, and personality that exist within the minds of the communicators. It is always present in communications. The context can be serious, humorous, formal, or strained. A skilled communicator will "check the mood" of other communicators to gauge appopropriateness of communications.

Communication Safety Alert

You will need to learn to keep your own psychological context separate from that of the patient and to focus on the patient's needs. Even if you are in a bad mood or are feeling frustrated, this cannot show during your nursing care or in conversations with patients and their family.

The *social* context includes the rules, standards, or norms that govern interpersonal communications relative to the status and nature of the relationship that exists between communicators. Whenever we communicate, we reveal something about the social rank of the relationship and the people with whom we communicate, just as we offer clues that help them define their relationship with us.[17]

The *spiritual* context refers to the meaning of life, hope, and purpose of existence for the communicators. Spirituality includes, but is not limited to, religious beliefs.

In a *professional* context, additional rules and norms will guide your behavior and communication choices. Within the professional context in health care, nurses communicate and work collaboratively with patients and other health disciplines to promote optimal health outcomes.

Element No. 10 Communication Risk Factors

Communication risk factors have the potential to distort clear communication by interfering with the exactness of the message.[17] This leads to misinterpretations that can create frustrations, negative feelings, and inaccurate clinical decision making.

Risk factors can occur at any point during communications. Table 2.2 provides some examples of the physical, psychological, physiological, and semantic types of risk factors in social and health-care settings.

Element No. 11: Patient-Safe Strategies

There are specific patient-safe communication strategies that can be used to overcome communication risk factors. For example, when a patient is anxious (risk factor), he or she cannot focus on communications. Through use of touch (patient-safe strategy), you can communicate care and concern and reduce the individual's anxiety level. The third ring of the transformational model contains patient-safe communication strategies.

Element No. 12: Transformation

Communication is transformational because individuals continue to grow and evolve biologically, psychologically, socially, culturally, and spiritually throughout their lives based on the outcomes of communication. Communication changes individuals from the people they were prior to the communication experience. Transformation is represented by the outer ring as an encapsulating outcome of the communication process as shown in Figure 2.5.

TABLE 2.2	Examples of Risk Factors in Social and Health-Care Settings	
Risk Factors	**Examples in Social Settings**	**Examples in Health-Care Settings**
Physical	Crowded room, noisy gathering, distasteful outfit, bizarre makeup	Alarms, overhead pages, lack of privacy, noisy hallways
Psychological	Bad mood, distraction by inner thoughts and stressors, stereotyping, bias, prejudices	Stress of illness, fear of the unknown, maladaptive coping responses, preconceived judgments
Physiological	Pain, anxiety, nervousness, twitch, having to go to the bathroom	Anxiety, acute pain, heavy sedation, cognitive or sensory impairment
Semantic	Intoxicated speech, monotone voice, heavy accent, English as second language	Slurred speech, accent, literacy level, illegible handwriting, spelling mistakes, abbreviations

Communication as Defined in the Transformational Model

Now that each of the elements of the transformational model has been defined, communication can be defined to include the critical components of effects and outcomes. Communication is:

- A goal-oriented, transformational interaction between two or more people
- Where verbal and nonverbal behavior is exchanged simultaneously to create common meaning
- And to create desired effects
- To achieve specific outcomes
- And attain transformation

CHAPTER SUMMARY

High-level communication competence includes four key components: effectiveness, appropriateness, sensitivity, and communicating in a way that saves face and maintains respect for self and others. The chapter introduced the transformational model as a practical and useful guide to attain high-level communication competence. The transformational model is especially useful to health-care providers because it is focused on the effects of messages and achieving desired transformational outcomes during communication.

BUILDING HIGH-LEVEL COMMUNICATION COMPETENCE

For additional exercises, visit DavisPlus at http://davisplus.fadavis.com

1. **Reflection.** Think about a conversation you had with someone recently that did not go the way you had expected. Write the scenario out and comment on the following: (1) which human need motivated your need to communicate, (2) the context of the situation and how your context may have differed from that of the person with whom you were comunicating, (3) the intended effect you were trying to create, (4) ability to create common meaning, (5) risk factors that interfered with the communication process, and (6) reasons why the desired outcome was not achieved.

2. **Practice.** Try assessing the context of a situation accurately. Look around you when you communicate—is the environment one that is conducive to having a conversation? Think about what would make the setting better. Consider situations in which you observed someone communicating out of context.

References

1. Spitzberg, B.H., Cupach, W. R. (1984). Interpersonal Communication Competence. Beverly Hills, Calif., Sage: 1984.
2. Parry, S.B. Just What is a Competency (And Why Should We Care?). Training 35:58-64, 1998.
3. Wilson, S.R., Sabee, C.M. Explicating Communication Competence as a Theoretical Term. In Greene, J.O. (ed.), Handbook of Communication and Social Interaction Skills, p. 50. Mahwah, N.J., Erlbaum: 2003.
4. Wiemann, J.M., Takai, J., Ota, H., et al.: A Relational Model of Communication Competence. In Kovacic, B. (ed.), Emerging Theories of Human Communication, Albany, N.Y., SUNY Press: 1997.
5. Gouran, D., Wiethoff, W.E., Doelger, J.A. Mastering Communication, 2nd ed. Boston, Allyn and Bacon: 1994.
6. Buber, M. I and Thou. New York, Scribners: 1958.
7. Beebe, S.A., Beebe, S., Redmond, M.V., et al.: Interpersonal Communication: Relating to Others, 4th ed. Toronto, Ontario, Pearson Education Canada: 2007.
8. Shannon, C.E., Weaver, E. The Mathematical Theory of Communication. Champaign, Ill., University of Illinois Press: 1949.
9. Leary, T. The Theory and Measurement Methodology of Interpersonal Communication. Psychiatry 18:147, 1955.
10. Foulger, D. 2004. Models of the Communication Process. http://foulger.info/davis/research/unifiedModelOfCommunication.htm Accessed Sept. 2009.
11. Schramm, W. How Communication Works. In Schramm, W. (ed.),The Process and Effects of Communication, pp. 3-26. Urbana, Ill., University of Illinois Press: 1954.
12. Barnlund, D.C. A Transactional Model of Communication. In Sereno, K.K., Mortensen, C.D. (eds). Foundations of Communication Theory. New York, Harper and Row: 1970.
13. Anderson, R., Ross, V. Questions of Communication: A Practical Introduction to Theory. New York, St. Martin's Press: 1994.
14. World Health Organization. Wilkinson, R., Marmot, M. (eds.), Social Determinants of Health: The Solid Facts, 2nd ed., 2003. http://www.euro.who.int/document/e81384.pdf Accessed November 2007.
15. Rubin, R.B., Perse, E.M., Barbato, C.A. Conceptualization and Measurement of Interpersonal Communication Motives. Human Communication Research 14:602-628, 1988.
16. Fogel, A., de Koeyer, I. Bellagamba, F., et al. The Dialogical Self in the First Two Years of Life: Embarking on a Journey of Discovery. Theory and Psychology 12:191-205, 2002.
17. Weaver, R.L. 1996. Understanding Interpersonal Communication, 7th ed. New York, Addison-Wesley Educational Publishers: 1996.
18. Dillard, J.P., Soloman, D.H., Palmer, M.T. Structuring the Concept of Relational Communication. Communication Monographs, 66:49-65, 1999.

Communicator Perceptions, Self-Concept, and Self-Esteem Within the Core of the Transformational Model

Learning Outcomes

Upon completion of this chapter, you will be able to:

1. Describe the relationship between self-concept, self-esteem, and perception in the communicators within the core of the transformational model of communication.
2. Explain the importance of understanding the unique perceptions of others.
3. Describe the purpose of the patient-safe strategy of perception checking.
4. Describe factors that influence our ability to perceive ourselves and others accurately.
5. Explain differences in the use of self-disclosure in social and professional relationships.
6. Describe how self-concept and self-esteem evolve throughout life.
7. Describe how self-esteem develops and affects communication and interpersonal relationships.
8. Identify patient-safe strategies to improve self-esteem.

Key Terms

Self-concept
Self-esteem
Perception
Closure
Superimpose
Select
Organize
Interpret
Attend
Attribution theory
Fish-and-water effect
Self-verification
Self-serving bias

Perception check
Belief
Value
Attitude
Reflected appraisal
Social comparison
Self-appraisal
Self-awareness
Disclosure
Johari window
Self-fulfilling prophecy
Fundamental attribution error

This chapter focuses on the communicators within the core of the transformational model and three unique characteristics of each communicator that affect every communication situation: self-concept, self-esteem, and perception. Self-concept is who the communicators think they are; self-esteem is what they think of themselves; and perception is how they perceive themselves, their world, and others within it. Self-concept, self-esteem, and perception are highlighted within the core of the transformational model as shown in Figure 3.1.

Having a better understanding of how you see yourself in terms of self-concept and self-esteem and how you see others in the world around you through your own perceptions helps you to appreciate the uniqueness of others when you communicate with them. This chapter covers the importance of self-awareness, perceiving others accurately, and developing sensitivity to the perspectives of others. *For an interactive version of this activity, visit DavisPlus at http://davisplus.fadavis.com*

How you answer the questions in the quiz depends on your perception of self. You communicate based on ideas of yourself and your perceptions. Self and perception are closely related and often difficult to separate because how you see others and the world around you depends on what you think of yourself.[1] To gain appreciation of the interrelatedness of self and perception in the communication process, think about two people communicating. Are there only two people involved or are there more? In every interpersonal communication you share with another person, at least six "people" are involved[2]:

1. The person you think you are
2. The person you think your partner is
3. The person your partner thinks s/he is
4. The person your partner thinks you are
5. The person you believe your partner thinks you are
6. The person your partner believes you think s/he is

In each statement, you can exchange the word "think" with the word "perceive" to begin to understand the importance of communicators' perceptions of themselves and others during any communication situation.

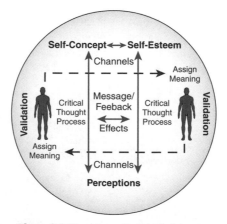

Figure 3.1 Transformational model core.

🧩 PERCEPTION AND HIGH-LEVEL COMMUNICATION COMPETENCE

Your perception is your reality, so that the world exists according to how you perceive it. The meanings we assign to words, objects, and events are based on our perceptions that come from within us and are influenced by who we are and our accumulated life experiences.

This same subjectivity and uniqueness of our perceptions applies in how we perceive others. George Clooney is sexy. Julia Roberts is beautiful. Brad Pitt is handsome. You either agree or disagree with each comment. You may have felt that different descriptions would be more accurate for these people. You may have thought of Clooney as a bachelor, Roberts as a redhead, and Pitt as a father. Your thoughts are unique, and you came to certain conclusions about these people through your ability to form perceptions.

Accepting that different realities exist simultaneously enhances our ability to be open, appreciative, and sensitive to the perspectives of others, which differ from our own. Individuals gain a sense of others' reality through the perspectives that are shared through thoughts, ideas, and opinions during communications.

Sensitivity to the perspectives of others is a high-level communication competency you will need to use in both personal and professional situations. The nurse enters the patient's world to see health-care experiences through the patient's eyes. By taking the patient's perspective into consideration, the nurse is able to plan interventions that are valued and meaningful for the patient. If the nurse does not take into consideration the patient's perspective, therapeutic regimes may not be followed, leading to patient harm.

Perception is a complex process, and we rarely think about how we are engaged in it. Most often we become attuned to our perceptions when we experience differences in perceptions with another person that have caused frustration or an argument. By understanding the perception process, you can improve your ability to communicate and have greater opportunity to create the intended effects and desired outcomes in interpersonal, nurse-patient, and interdisciplinary relationships.

The Perception Process

Perception is the process of gathering information and giving it meaning. We gather information through our senses. There are three stages in the perception process: selection, organization, and interpretation.

Selection

Because our senses are continually bombarded with stimuli, we are selective about the stimuli we choose to focus on in any given moment. We select according to various characteristics of the stimuli. Stimuli that are intense to our senses, such as a loud burst of laughter or a brightly colored outfit, will receive our attention immediately. Repetition or annoyance also attracts our attention, such as someone tapping a pen on the desk. Our motives and desires can also heighten our attention to specific stimuli in the environment. As an example, a nurse will be more aware of the signs and symptoms of hypoglycemia after administering insulin.

Organization

After selecting, we begin to arrange the stimuli in meaningful ways to make sense of them. We organize stimuli by determining generalities first and then fitting the stimuli into categories. Our classification of stimuli into categories is dependent upon our personality, acquired knowledge, and past experiences and tends to follow a common framework[3-5]:

- Physical (beautiful or ugly, short or tall, small or large)
- Similarity (are like my friends or not, dress like I do or not, are of my culture or not)
- Role or social position (teacher, police officer, colleague)
- Interaction (outgoing or shy, friendly or unfriendly, pleasant or obnoxious)
- Psychological (happy or sad, nervous or calm, insecure or confident)
- Expected behavior (how to dress, when to talk and when to listen, how to eat with proper table manners)

We also use closure to help us organize information. Look at Figure 3.2. Do you see a triangle and a square rather than a series of unconnected lines? The process of filling in gaps between pieces of information is called *closure*. From a minimum of cues we can put together a fairly complete picture, making sense of the available information through closure. Nevertheless, when we use closure, we may not form accurate perceptions upon which to base subsequent decisions.

Communication Safety Alert

The risk of harmful events increases when health-care providers use closure to "fill in the blanks" for patients. Although it may take patients time to tell their health history, and they may pause and stumble over words or not know the words to use, listen to the story in its entirety from their perspective, and do not fill in the blanks. Appropriate health-care decisions and clinical judgments are based on accurate communication with patients.

In addition, we also organize by *superimposing*. Superimpose means to *place a familiar structure* on the stimuli/information. Look at Figure 3.3 and determine if you can perceive the words. If you perceived this to be Tylenol tablets, you have superimposed. You have created meaningful words from an assemblage of letters of the alphabet. This same principle applies to our perceptions of people. When we have an incomplete picture of someone, we impose a pattern of behavior or structure to help us understand who they are.

Communication Safety Alert

Superimposing when a doctor's order is not written legibly can lead to medication and treatment errors that cause patient harm. Superimposing a particular stereotype on a patient, such as "men are more tolerant of pain than women," can lead to inappropriate treatment.

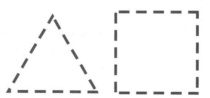

Figure 3.2 This example represents the concept of closure.

Tylnol tblt

Figure 3.3 This example represents the concept of superimposing.

Interpretation

The final stage of the perception process is interpretation. Once we have selected and organized stimuli into categories, we are ready to interpret what the information means. When we interpret, we assign meaning to the stimuli from our senses that are based on our own unique reality.

Our Motivation to Perceive Others

It is a part of our human nature that we are motivated to perceive others. We are motivated to anticipate the behavioral response of others to our communications because we have a preference for a reality that is predictable and stable.[6] As an example, think of your initial week of class when you first started your nursing program. In all likelihood you were observing your new classmates and instructors. You were forming perceptions of who they were. Until we get to know individuals better by observing them, interacting with them, and learning more about who they are, we experience feelings of uncertainty and ambiguity.[7]

Behavioral acts constitute the building blocks of perceiving others.[8] The behaviors individuals express when they interact with others, consciously or unconsciously, verbally or nonverbally, are a direct result of their perceptions and their sense of self. We interpret and assign meaning to behavior we hear and observe and make inferences about the motives of others, their personalities, and other traits based on our observations.[9] If we can gain information about individuals and reduce uncertainty, we can predict their reactions and behaviors to our communications, adapt our behaviors and communication strategies accordingly, and maximize the likelihood of fulfilling our desired outcomes.[10] Our motivation to perceive others is illustrated in Figure 3.4.

Every day, to achieve our desired outcomes, we adjust our communication behavior based on our perceptions of others and our predictions of how they will respond to us. Suppose it is your intention to provide discharge patient teaching. You walk into the room and observe that the patient is in tears. The emotional issues must be acknowledged and addressed first before the patient can focus on learning self-care.

Factors That Influence the Ability to Perceive Others Accurately

Attribution theory explains how we ascribe specific motives and causes to the behaviors of others.[7] It helps us interpret what people do and why they are doing it. Developing the most logical explanation for the behavior of others is the goal of the attribution process.[7]

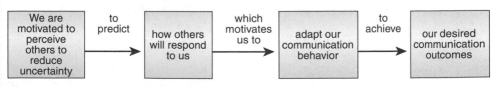

Figure 3.4 Our motivation to perceive others.

Our ability to perceive others can be highly inaccurate, however. Examples of how we inaccurately attribute motives and causes of behavior to others in our personal and professional life include the following:

1. *We form perceptions according to stereotypes.* We form broad generalizations about groups of people and conclude that all who belong to the group are the same. When we stereotype, we obscure the uniqueness of the individual.

2. *We cling to first impressions, even if they are wrong.* We label people by what our senses tell us the first time (for example, "He's happy-go-lucky," "She's so serious.") Once we form an opinion of someone, we tend to hold fast to it and make any conflicting information fit our opinion.[3]

3. *We tend to assume that others think and behave as we do.* If we like quiet while we are studying, we believe others do as well. Not only do we assume that others believe as we do, we have a tendency to conclude that there is something wrong with people who do not think like we do. As a nurse, it is important that you understand that others do not think, do not feel, and are not motivated to act in the same way as you.

4. *We tend to favor negative impressions over positive ones.* When we are aware of the positive and negative qualities of an individual, the negative qualities have a greater influence on how we perceive and assign meaning to the characteristics of the individual.

5. *We are influenced by our expectations.* We expect people to behave in a certain way. When they behave outside our set of expectations, we may form negative impressions of them. Understanding the influence of culture and other factors on how people behave will make it easier for you to accept variations in expected behaviors and to interpret the motives and behaviors of others more accurately.

6. *We judge others more harshly than ourselves, given the same situation.* This tendency is called the self-serving bias. It is our human nature to enhance ourself. For example, we tend to believe we are more trustworthy and moral than others.[11] The self-serving bias is a mechanism through which we maintain our positive beliefs in ourself.[12] When others have misfortunes, we blame the problem on their personal qualities; when we have misfortunes, we find explanations outside ourselves.[13]

7. *We take credit for success while denying responsibility for failure.* This is another expression of the self-serving bias.[12] We tend to say we attained something when a task outcome is successful but blame circumstances or others for failed task outcomes.[11]

8. *We are more likely to believe that people are to blame when they make mistakes than to believe that mistakes made were beyond their control.* This perception error is called the fundamental attribution error.[13] We believe that the cause of a problem or a mistake is something personally controllable; therefore, we attribute the mistake to an individual's personal qualities or weakness of character.[7] As you will read in Unit 3, however, there are many factors that cause mistakes that have little to do with individual character.

PATIENT-SAFE COMMUNICATION STRATEGY TO IMPROVE PERCEIVING OTHERS ACCURATELY: PERCEPTION CHECKING

Perception checking is a patient-safe communication strategy that helps us interpret the verbal and nonverbal behavior of others with greater accuracy and is a mechanism by which we create common meaning. It is a means to determine if your perceptions are correct, rather than relying on assumptions and the assigned meaning associated with your perception process that is influenced by who you are and involves just you. Adler[3] suggests that the perception check includes three components:

1. A description of the behavior you noticed
2. Two possible interpretations of the behavior
3. A request for clarification about how to interpret the behavior.

Consider the following nursing example. You are assigned to care for a first-day postoperative patient. The patient denies pain when you ask her to rate her pain on a 10-point scale. You see, however, that she is on the verge of tears. You check perception with her: "I know you denied pain when I asked, but I can see that you have tears in your eyes [behavior]. Are you having pain [first interpretation], or has something happened to upset you [second interpretation]? I need to know what is happening here so that I can help you [request for clarification]." In nursing, perception checking is used to ensure we are interpreting our patients' behavior accurately.

The goal of perception checking is mutual understanding and a cooperative approach to communication. It signals an attitude of respect and concern for the other person.[3] Weaver[13] describes that perception checking improves communication and relationships because interactions between individuals:

1. Become grounded on perceptions that are more accurate because perceptions are tested through actual interaction
2. Become better adapted to each individual because each has a better understanding of the needs of the other
3. Become less open to chance because there is less guessing about the person and the message
4. Are at less risk for breakdown from misinterpretation and misperceptions

The remainder of the chapter addresses the importance of self-perception in communication with others. Specifically, it discusses how self-concept and self-esteem develop and the effect of both on communication in interpersonal relationships.

✛ PERCEIVING OURSELVES: THE SELF IN COMMUNICATIONS

Our sense of self is derived from our self-concept and our self-esteem. Through self-concept you *describe* who you are; through self-esteem you *evaluate* who you are. Both influence how you approach, respond to, and perceive others and the messages they share with you during communications.

How Self-Concept Develops

Throughout a person's life, the concept of self evolves. Self-concept refers to our definitions of self, filtered through our perception of who we think we are. We use subjective labels to define who we are from many perspectives. For example, you may define your sense of self through personal descriptors such as tall, outgoing, or reliable. You may define yourself through the social roles you play, such as parent, spouse, friend, and student nurse. You may define yourself through groups to which you belong, such as singer in a choir or fitness club member. Culturally, you may define yourself as Muslim or Jewish. You may describe yourself as a citizen of a country. You may define yourself through the possessions you have, such as a luxury car or expensive jewelry. Collectively, the sum of all of our perceptions of self allows us to know who we are by experiencing ourselves in relation to others and our significant life events.

Who you are is reflected in your personal values, attitudes, and beliefs. These are all *learned responses* from your life experiences that shape self-concept and behavior.[7]

- A *value* is an enduring concept of good or bad, right and wrong. Values are formed by your interpersonal relationships beginning with the messages you received as children from your parents. For example, you may have learned to value education as something good, cheating as something bad. Values are more resistant to change than either attitudes or beliefs.
- An *attitude* represents your likes and dislikes. Attitude is your learned response, either favorable or unfavorable, to a person, object, event, or idea.
- *Beliefs* are the ways in which you create reality through determining if something is true or false. Beliefs are built from what you have learned through previous experiences.

The development of self-concept is a complex process. We are not born with a concept of self; it is accumulated through our interactions with the world.[15] This evolution is influenced by four key factors: reflected appraisal, social comparisons, cultural and societal influence, and self-appraisal.

Reflected Appraisals

In the early 1900s, sociologist George Cooley introduced the theory that self-concept is developed by seeing ourselves through a looking glass.[16] The looking glass, or reflected appraisal, is the mechanism for learning who we are by the way others respond to us and treat us. In other words, the way we believe others perceive us is the way we perceive ourselves.[17]

To the extent that you receive supportive messages, you perceive yourself as confident and capable, and you appreciate and value yourself. To the extent that you receive messages of criticism, you perceive yourself as less valuable and capable.[18]

Bergner and Holmes[19] describe four requirements that must be met before a reflected appraisal will be regarded important enough to affect self-concept:

1. The person offering the appraisal must be someone perceived as competent to do so.
2. The appraisal must be reasonable in terms of an individual's self-belief.
3. The appraisal must come from someone who has earned the individual's confidence.
4. Appraisals that are consistent and numerous are more persuasive than appraisals that are single events.

Social Comparisons

We also develop self-concept by evaluating ourselves in terms of how we compare with others. Social comparison refers to the process through which people come to know themselves by evaluating their knowledge, values, attitudes, and skills in comparison with others. In most cases, we try to compare ourselves with those in our peer group or with those with whom we are similar. In the nursing profession, for example, you will compare yourself to other nurses on the patient care unit to see if you are as skilled, knowledgeable, or compassionate. You gain additional perspective and self-definitions when you draw comparisons.

Societal and Cultural Influence
Through your upbringing, you were influenced by the traditions of your culture, the norms of your community, and expectations of society. These influences became part of who you are. For example, a societal norm for zero tolerance for impaired drivers may shape your beliefs, values, and attitudes about designated drivers.

Self-Appraisal
Your self-concept is influenced through self-appraisal. You react to and evaluate your own behavior, quirks, and beliefs. For example, people may tell you that you are confident and outgoing, yet you know that you are actually quite shy and nervous around people you do not know. Collectively, reflected appraisals, social comparisons, societal and cultural influence, and self-appraisal help to develop our identity and self-concept.

Characteristics of the Self-Concept
Now that you have a better idea of how your self-concept has developed, we can take a closer look at some of its particular characteristics. These include resistance to change and the self-fulfilling prophecy.

Resistance to Change
Self-concept is highly resistant to change.[6] This holds true even when a new concept of self would be more favorable. Once we fasten onto a concept of self, whether positive or negative, we have a tendency to cling to it and will seek out people who confirm our perceptions of self-concept. This human behavior is called self-verification and is based on a social psychology theory developed by William Swann,[6] which suggests that people want to be known and understood by others according to their firmly held beliefs and feelings about themselves. According to Swann, there is an uncomfortable disorientation in the sense of self that occurs when we are redefined by others in a new way. We work to ensure the stability of our self-concept and to be defined by others consistent with our own views and perception of self. When faced with information that contradicts our self-concept, we are faced with a decision. We can ponder the new information, accept it, and grow and evolve through a transformational experience or remain steadfast in our self-view and discard the new information.

Self-Fulfilling Prophecy
The self-concept is such a powerful force that it not only determines how you see yourself in the present but also influences your future behavior and that of others.[3] This characteristic has been termed the *self-fulfilling prophecy*. Conceptualized by Robert Merton,[20] the self-fulfilling prophecy is like a prediction or a possibility of an outcome that comes true as a result of a person's conscious or unconscious actions. There are two types of prophecies. The first is the *self-imposed prophecy*. This occurs when an individual creates a prediction or an expectation of an outcome, and the individual changes behavior to make the prophecy come true.

The second is the *Pygmalion effect,* whereby your beliefs and expectations of another cause the behavior of that individual to occur.[21] You consciously or subconsciously treat people according to your expectations, and how you treat them causes them to act according to your expectations. The Pygmalion effect involves four key principles:

1. We form expectations of people or events
2. We communicate the expectations through various cues

3. People tend to respond to the cues by adjusting their behavior to match them

4. The result is that the expectation comes true

In health care, we see the negative effects of the self-fulfilling prophecy when a patient with a poor self-concept says, "I'll never be able to remember anything you are telling me about my discharge instructions." The nurse responds, "We will go over the instructions together, and I can review with you any areas you feel are still unclear." The patient states, "Don't bother, I just know I'll never get it right." In this example, the patient has created the prophecy that he will not understand the instructions, and by his conscious and subconscious behaviors he will make the prophecy come true, unless the nurse communicates effectively to boost his confidence.

Factors That Affect Our Ability to Perceive Our Self Accurately

It is common to have inaccurate perceptions of ourselves. This tends to occur because individuals have difficulty in perceiving their own behavior objectively.[6,8,22] Research shows that in comparisons between self-ratings and judgments about behavior provided by peers and acquaintances, individuals' self-perceptions are less accurate in comparison with the perceptions of others.[8,22] These studies concluded that individuals become so accustomed to their own behavioral patterns that they become relatively unaware of them. Kolar and colleagues[22] have described this behavior as the "fish-and-water effect" in that "it is difficult for humans to detect their own stable behavioral tendencies, for essentially the same reason that fish are said to find it difficult to detect water."

Strategies to Improve Perceiving Ourselves More Accurately

The ability to perceive ourselves with accuracy means that we have self-awareness. Self-awareness is the extent to which you know yourself accurately and is the total sum of your perceptions of yourself.[14] The main reason to develop a high level of self-awareness is because you must understand your own uniqueness before you can fully appreciate the uniqueness of others. From knowing your own frame of reference, you can gauge and predict others better by how similar or different they are from you. This knowledge will help you plan how to communicate with others more effectively, appropriately, and sensitively. In nursing, it is extremely important to have a high level of self-awareness to recognize the differences between your personal health beliefs and those of your patients. You need to appreciate differences in perspectives and to develop effective patient-valued interventions. Developing a high level of self-awareness is not easy, nor is it something you can do completely on your own. You need feedback from others to increase self-awareness.

Increasing Self-Awareness—Looking Through the Johari Window

A theoretical framework that describes how you can increase self-awareness through feedback is the Johari Window created by Joseph Luft and Harry Ingham.[23] It describes self-awareness through the four selves: the open self, blind self, hidden self, and unknown self. The four selves are represented as four connected windowpanes, as shown in Figure 3.5.

1. *Open self:* The open self represents behaviors, thoughts, feelings, attitudes, motivations, and aspirations that are known by you and others. The extent to which you let others know about you dictates the size of this quadrant. Within interpersonal relationships that you have had for years, this quadrant is large. When you meet someone for the first time, this quadrant is very small.

	Known to Self	Not Known to Self
Known to Others	**Open Self** Information about yourself that you and others know	**Blind Self** Information about yourself that you do not know but others do know
Not Known to Others	**Hidden Self** Information about yourself that you do know but others do not know	**Unknown Self** Information about yourself that neither you nor others know

Figure 3.5 The Johari window.

2. *Blind self:* This quadrant represents the things people know about you but that you do not know about yourself. You may feel you are a good conversationalist, but other people consistently find you ramble from topic to topic. People who have a large blind self quadrant can be frustrating to be around because they have little idea about how they come across to others.
3. *Hidden self:* In this quadrant the hidden self represents all that you know of yourself but purposely keep hidden from others. This may be embarrassments you do not want to share with others, or it may be information that you hold back until you know the person better.
4. *Unknown self:* The unknown self represents the truths about yourself that neither you nor others know. In the most complex sense, this refers to repressed memories. In a practical sense, it refers to your life as it evolves throughout your lifetime.

The main theme of the Johari Window is that self-awareness can be increased by getting to know your blind self through eliciting feedback from others. Your family, close friends, other students, and nursing faculty will each see you differently and may give different feedback. You are all of these selves.

The following are methods you can use to increase your self-awareness:

- Listen, really listen, to others.
- Seek out information about yourself to increase self-awareness because others will perceive you with greater accuracy than you perceive yourself.

Self-Disclosure

Self-disclosure is sharing information that others would not normally know or discover.[24] In order for communication to be considered self-disclosing, it must contain personal information about the sender; the sender must communicate this information; and another person must be an intended target.[25] You can learn more about yourself and develop increased self-awareness through self-disclosure. When you self-disclose, others learn about who you are at a deeper, more personal, level. They are able to provide you with accurate feedback on who you are because they know your uniqueness and how you see the world around you. They share their observations, insights, and perspectives of you, and self-awareness increases.

Within social relationships, when you self-disclose to someone, the other will also disclose. This is known as the norm of reciprocity.[26] Knowing more about each other reduces uncertainty and ambiguity in how you each will respond during communications; as a result, communication and relationships improve. Rosenfeld[27] suggests people disclose for a variety of reasons:

- Unload—vent, get something off their chest
- Self-clarification—clarify beliefs, opinions, thoughts, attitudes
- Self-validation—elicit confirmation about a self-belief

Other reasons individuals disclose personal information include:

- Impression formation—means to market oneself to others during a job interview or to develop a romantic relationship[28]
- Relationship maintenance—relationships must be nourished by self-disclosure[29]
- Societal influence—a means of helping others, such as self-help groups[30]
- Health needs—express one's health beliefs and behaviors that may have contributed to the current health state

Guidelines for Disclosure in Nurse-Patient Relationships: A Patient-Safe Communication Strategy

Nurses encourage patients to disclose personal information. Access to patient information helps the health-care team determine health status, behavior, beliefs, resources, and coping mechanisms to guide accurate clinical decision making and to implement appropriate patient-specific interventions. Nurses do not disclose in the nurse-patient relationship in the same way they do in private interpersonal relationships. Disclosure in relationships with patients must be purposeful. Purposeful disclosure is a patient-safe therapeutic response that can increase the patient's comfort during a procedure or during the health assessment. For example, the nurse may disclose the following during a health assessment when it appears the patient is stressed trying to balance work and home life: "Sometimes I am so busy that I forget to take the time to just relax and have some quiet time alone. Does this sometimes happen to you as well?" The patient would then feel encouraged to agree or disagree and know it is safe to add specific details from his own perspective. Purposeful self-disclosure by the nurse may promote honesty and openness for the patient but never burdens the patient with the nurses' problems.[31] Figure 3.6 provides a comparison of disclosure and outcomes in interpersonal and nurse-patient relationships.

Self-Esteem: How Much Do You Like and Accept Yourself?

Self-esteem is defined as the value or worth you place on yourself.[7] It is derived from how well you like and accept yourself. Self-esteem is based on self-respect and the respect you receive from significant others.[32] Self-respect means you have a sense of competence, confidence, mastery, achievement, independence, and freedom. Social comparisons can influence your sense of self-esteem because you draw conclusions of your value by how you stand in relation to others. Reflected appraisals also influence your self-esteem based on the feedback you receive from others. Your self-esteem affects your ability to be sensitive to others, manifests in how you typically communicate, and affects how you will perceive messages.[7] In other words, it can affect your ability to communicate with high-level competency. High or low levels of self-esteem lead to differences in how individuals develop and maintain interpersonal relationships with significant others.

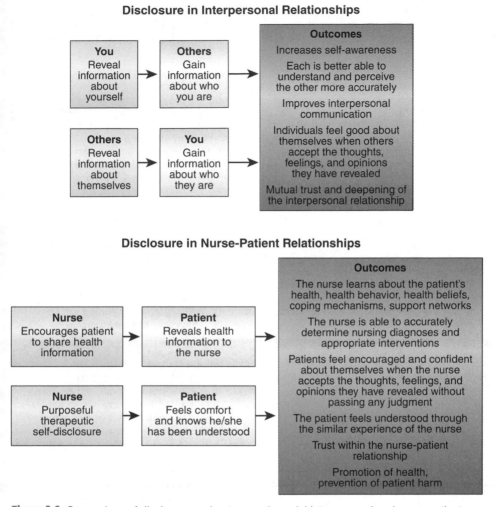

Figure 3.6 Comparison of disclosure and outcomes in social interpersonal and nurse-patient relationships.

How Levels of Esteem Affect Communication and Interpersonal Relationships

The communication styles of people based on self-esteem are rooted in family development theory.[33] Low self-esteem exacts a high price on individual and interpersonal relationships. With low self-esteem, communication is indirect, vague, and dishonest. The person responds to others fearfully and feels tension and stress. The result of low self-esteem is loneliness and isolation.

The person with high self-esteem responds to others receptively, really listens to what others are saying, and treats others with respect. The person can ask for advice and help from others but also can make decisions. A person with high self-esteem is not afraid to fail and can learn from mistakes. Increasing self-esteem in ourselves and others is a prerequisite for high-level communication competency.

Strategies to Improve Self-Esteem

How can we overcome our innate resistance to change to allow ourselves to grow and develop positive self-esteem? Try the following techniques outlined in Table 3.1.

TABLE 3.1 Developing Positive Self-Esteem	
To Increase Your Self-Esteem:	
Use affirmations and positive statements	These statements help reinforce positive aspects of your personality and experience. Every day, you can boost your sense of self-esteem by saying positive things to yourself, such as "I am a caring person."
Visualization exercises	List the things you would like to experience. Construct the statements as if you were already enjoying the situations you list, beginning each statement with "I am...." Visualize each situation, and get into the habit of repeating this process several times a day.
Tune out your negative critic	Instead, think of a situation you handled well or something of which you are really proud.
To Increase the Self-Esteem of Others:	
Define clear and realistic goals	People with low self-esteem often tend to over-generalize and think in nonspecific ways. They may say, "I just want to be happy." Respond by asking for more specifics, "What does happiness mean to you?" Turning a general, nonspecific feeling into a goal toward which to work promotes the path to improved self-esteem.
Give positive feedback	Giving honest praise to people for what they have achieved bolsters their self-esteem. However, the praise must be honest and true to the person's accomplishment.

CHAPTER SUMMARY

The focus of this chapter was on the communicators within the core of the transformational model and the unique components of perception and self that they bring to each communication situation. The chapter began with the perception process and described how individuals form perceptions and assign meaning to what they hear and observe from their own unique perspective. Although we all go through the same perception process, no two individuals will perceive words, events, or people the same way. The chapter also focused on the self in communications, which includes self-concept and self-esteem. Development of self-concept is a complex process that is influenced by reflected appraisals, social comparisons, societal and cultural influences, and self-appraisals. Finally, the chapter focused on self-esteem. Having a high level of self-esteem and self-awareness, and understanding the perceptual variances that interplay during communications, will help you to communicate with high-level competency in your personal and professional life.

 BUILDING HIGH-LEVEL COMMUNICATION COMPETENCE

For additional exercises, visit DavisPlus at http://davisplus.fadavis.com

1. **Reflection.** "Who Are You" exercise.[7] The responses will help you begin to explore your perceptions and sense of self.

   Who Are You?

   Ask yourself the question, "Who are you?" Ask yourself 10 times. Write each of your responses on a piece of paper.

   Did you find this a hard exercise? Did you have to stop and really think about who you are? This exercise provides an opportunity for you to self-perceive and to develop greater self-awareness.

2. **Critical Thinking.** Read the following scenario and answer the questions:

   The nurse is taking a health history and asks the patient to describe his symptoms. He is vague in describing how long he has had the symptoms by saying, "The pain started recently, but it's actually been going on for a long time."

A. Using the three components of perception checking, how would you clarify the patient's description of the duration of his symptoms?

   The nurse then asks if the patient has any allergies. He replies that he has no allergies but had some redness from the tape used during his last hospitalization. The nurse informs the patient that he has described an allergy to tape. The patient remarks, "OK, now I know."

B. Where did creating common meaning of the term "allergy" occur in this situation?

   Later, the patient tells his wife, "My nurse thinks I am an idiot because I didn't know that I had an allergy to tape. Maybe I am an idiot. Maybe I just won't say anything at all when she asks me questions."

C. How might the nurse have informed the patient that redness from tape is an allergy that was interpreted by the patient as "the nurse thinks I am an idiot"? How could the nurse respond in a more sensitive way?

D. What type of self-fulfilling prophecy has occurred: the self-imposing prophecy or the Pygmalion effect?

   Answers are located at the back of the book.

References

1. Hybels, S., Weaver R.L. Communicating Effectively, 8th ed. McGraw-Hill, New York: 2007.
2. Barnlund, D.C. Toward a Meaning-Centered Philosophy of Communication. Journal of Communication 12:202, 1962.
3. Adler, R.B., Rosenfeld, L.B., Proctor R.F., et al. Interplay: The Process of Interpersonal Communication. Don Mills, Ontario, Oxford University Press: 2006, pp. 68-92.
4. DeVito, J.A. The Interpersonal Communication Book, 11th ed. Toronto, Ontario, Pearson Education: Canada: 2007.
5. Andersen, P.A. Nonverbal Communication: Forms and Functions. Palo Alto, Calif., Mayfield: 1999.
6. Swann, W.B. Self-Verification: Bringing Social Reality Into Harmony With the Self. In Suls, J., Greenwald, A.G. (Eds.), Psychological Perspectives on the Self, vol. 2. Hillsdale, N.J., Erlbaum: 1983, pp. 33-66.
7. Beebe, S.A., Beebe, S.J., Redmond, M.V., et al. Interpersonal Communication, 4th ed. Toronto, Ontario, Pearson Education Canada: 2007.
8. Gosling, S.D., John, O.P., Craik, K.H., et al. Do People Know How They Behave? Self-Reported Act Frequencies Compared With On-Line Codings by Observers. Journal of Personality and Social Psychology 74:1337-1349, 1998.
9. Hinton, P.R. The Psychology of Interpersonal Perception. New York, Routledge: 1993.
10. Berger, C.R., Bradac, J.J. Language and Social Knowledge. Baltimore, Edward Arnold: 1982.
11. Sedikides, C., Campbell, W.K., Reeder, G. D., et al. The Self-Serving Bias in Relational Context. Journal of Personality and Social Psychology 74:378-386, 1998.
12. Miller, D. T., Ross, M. Self-Serving Biases in Attribution of Causality: Fact or Fiction? Psychological Bulletin 82:213-225, 1975
13. Floyd, K. Attributions for nonnverbal expressions of liking and disliking: The extended self-serving bias. Western Journal of Communication, 64, 385-404, 2000.
14. Weaver, R.L. Understanding Interpersonal Communication. 7th ed. New York, Addison-Wesley: 1996.
15. Rosenblith, J.F. In the Beginning: Development From Conception to Age Two. Newbury Park, Calif., Sage: 1992
16. Cooley, G.H. Human Nature and the Social Order. New York, Scribner's: 1912.
17. Van Wagner, K. The Reflected Appraisal Process http://psychology.about.com/od/rindex/g/reflectapp.htm Accessed November, 2007.
18. Felson, R.B. Reflected Appraisal and the Development of Self. Social Psychology Quarterly 48:71-78, 1985.
19. Bergner, R.M., Holmes, J.R. Self-Concepts and Self-Concept Change: A Status Dynamic Approach. Psychotherapy: Theory, Research, Practice, Training 37:36-44, 2000.
20. Merton, R.K. Social Theory and Social Structure. New York, Free Press: 1968.
21. Rosenthal. R., Jacobson, L. Pygmalion in the Classroom. New York, Holt, Rhinehart and Winston: 1968.
22. Kolar, D.W., Funder, D.C., Colvin R.C. Comparing the Accuracy of Personality Judgments by the Self and Knowledgeable Others. Journal of Personality 64:311-337, 1996.
23. Luft, J., Ingham, H. The Johari Window: A Graphic Model of Interpersonal Awareness. Proceedings of the Western Training Laboratory in Group Development. Los Angeles, UCLA: 1955.
24. Jourard, S.M. A Study of Self-Disclosure. Scientific American 198:77-82, 1958.
25. Cozby, P.C. Self-Disclosure: A Literature Review. Psychological Bulletin 79:73-91, 1973.
26. Solanoc, H., Dunnam, M. Two's Company: Self-Disclosure and Reciprocity in Triads Versus Dyads. Social Psychology Quarterly 48:2, 1985.
27. Rosenfeld, L.B. Overview of the Ways Privacy, Secrecy, and Disclosure are Balanced in Today's Society. In Petronio, S. (ed.), Balancing the Secrets of Private Disclosures. Mahwah, N.J., Lawrence Erlbaum: 2000, pp. 3-17.
28. Stiles, W.B., Waltz, N.C., Schroeder, M.A.B., et al. Attractiveness and Disclosure in Initial Encounters of Mixed-Sex Dyads. Journal of Social and Personal Relationships 13:303-312, 1996.
29. Rosenfeld, L.B., Bowen, G.L. Marital Disclosure and Marital Satisfaction: Direct-Effect Versus Interaction-Effect Models. Western Journal of Speech Communication 55:69-84, 1991.
30. Priest, P.J., Dominic, J.R. Pulp Pulpits: Self-Disclosure on "Donahue." Journal of Communication 44:74, 1994.
31. Keltner, N.L., Schwecke, L.H., Bostrom, C.E. Psychiatric Nursing, St. Louis, Mosby: 1999.
32. Maslow, A.H. A Theory of Human Motivation. Psychological Review 50:370-396, 1943.
33. Satir, V. The New Peoplemaking. Mountainview, Calif., Science and Behavior Books: 1988.

Creating Common Meaning to Attain Transformational Outcomes

Learning Outcomes

Upon completion of this chapter, you will be able to:

1. Explain how to create common meaning to attain positive transformational outcomes.
2. Describe how to use verbal language and nonverbal behavior to convey messages effectively.
3. Identify appropriate channels to send messages to another.
4. Describe the listening process and risk factors that interfere with listening.
5. Describe patient-safe communication strategies that improve the ability to listen effectively.

Key Terms

Active listening
Blocking responses
Connotative
Denotative
Empathy
Paraphrasing

Paralanguage
Proxemics
Gestures
Eye contact
Facial expressions
Touch

This chapter focuses on how we create common meaning with others so as to create positive transformations and positive outcomes in health-care situations. By establishing mutually shared understanding between communicators, we can avoid miscommunications through misinterpretations and misunderstandings and, ultimately, avoid patient harm. Transformational outcomes are attained through high-level communication involving purposeful conveyance, channeling and reception of messages to create common meaning between communicators. The chapter describes factors that pose risk to listening effectively and examines patient-safe communication strategies that can improve the effectiveness of listening. *For an interactive version of this activity, visit DavisPlus at http://davisplus.fadavis.com*

This chapter specifically focuses on how high-level communicators use verbal language and nonverbal behavior to convey messages effectively, select channels to send messages, and receive and respond to messages through the listening process and effective listening responses.

CONVEYING MESSAGES THROUGH VERBAL LANGUAGE

Language is the primary vehicle through which we convey verbal messages to share our sense of the world with others.[1] Words are symbols of reality and arbitrarily represent something. They are not complete until they acquire meaning that is assigned by communicators. Consider the word "cat." The word does not look like a cat or sound like a cat; rather it is a collection of letters of the alphabet that translates into a word that symbolically indicates a cat. The dictionary definition of a word provides the *denotative meaning*. In this instance, the denotative meaning is a feline with four legs, whiskers, and a tail.

When we see or hear the word cat, however, we call on our personal images, past experiences, and feelings that help us assign meaning to this word. The inclusion of this information in our definition constitutes the *connotative meaning* of a word. Therefore, the word cat may mean a favored pet that is fluffy and purrs or a barnyard cat that is mangy and hisses. The connotative meaning of words represents our personal and subjective meaning as influenced by our unique perceptions.

In conversations throughout an average day, we use approximately 2000 words. Of these words, the 500 we use most often have over 14,000 dictionary definitions, which makes creating common meaning difficult in and of itself.[2] Imagine the increased complexity of creating common meaning when you add in the different connotations of words that exist as a result of individual perceptions and life experiences. Because meanings are in people and not in the words themselves, words are often misunderstood in conversation. As described by Weaver[3]:

1. What you hear is not necessarily the message conveyed. Even though words may be carefully selected through critical thought processing, this does not guarantee they will be interpreted as intended.
2. Meanings are negotiated. High-level communicators provide feedback regarding their understanding of a message. There may be a large gap between the intended meaning of the sender and the initial interpretation of the message by the receiver. Communicators clarify and verify the meaning of a message by providing feedback to narrow the gap and negotiate common meaning.
3. Meanings are personal and may not ever be totally revealed or shared during communications.

4. Confusion, misunderstanding, and conflict in relationships most often result from differences in meanings.
5. Awareness and sensitivity in interpersonal, nurse-patient, and interdisciplinary communications are important. Do not assume that words mean the same thing to different individuals; clarify meanings by asking questions; actively seek feedback to help others interpret messages within your intended meaning.

It is important to understand that words can evoke unpredictable effects or responses, reactions, and results in people. Individuals react to words according to the meanings they have assigned. Therefore, high-level communicators will purposefully select the words to convey their messages depending on their perception of how others will respond to and interpret the message. Consider the following examples of a simple request to "shut the door"[4]:

1. Close the door.
2. Can you close the door?
3. Would you please close the door?
4. It might help if you would close the door.
5. Would you mind terribly if I asked that you close the door?
6. Did you forget the door?
7. How about a bit less breeze?
8. It's getting pretty drafty in here.
9. I don't want the cat to get out.

We use critical thought processing to make careful adaptations to ensure our communications are appropriate for the context of the given situation and for the individuals to whom we direct the message. High-level communicators avoid sending ambiguous verbal messages.

Conveying Messages Using Words Clearly and Precisely

Words follow a continuum from concrete to abstract. The more concrete words are, the greater their clarity and ability to be understood easily by others as intended. Concrete words tend to be denotative, therefore less open to misinterpretation. Abstract words tend to be more connotative and more open to misinterpretation. Words such as "intramuscular" and "Demerol" are more concrete than abstract words such as "route" and "pain medication." In the latter examples, the word route is vague and can be interpreted to mean orally, subcutaneously, intramuscularly, or intravenously. Pain medication can mean anything from Tylenol to Demerol. Communicators use critical thought processing to select words and send messages that are precise. This increases the probability that the message can be interpreted by others as intended.

Avoid Ambiguous Verbal Messages

Every day, we send and receive ambiguous verbal messages. Think of the statement, "Run the patient down to X-ray." Does this mean the patient is unstable and *needs* to go quickly to X-ray, or is it slang for "take the patient to X-ray"? Can the patient walk, or should the patient be transported by wheelchair? Misinterpretations are possible due to the use of ambiguous slang words in the English language.

Other times we choose ambiguous verbal messages deliberately. For example, we have all had uncomfortable moments when someone asks us if we could help them in some particular way and we are not interested in doing so. Rather than communicating with a clear statement of non-interest, we may reply by being noncommittal: "I am not sure," "I'll have to check," or "I think I already have something planned."

Sometimes we use generalizations or stereotypes, which also contribute to ambiguous verbal messages. *"Every physician* should take a course in handwriting" or *"All nurses* need to work on patient confidentiality." In reality, not every doctor in the world has unreadable handwriting, and not every nurse worldwide breeches confidentiality.

The use of tag questions also sends ambiguous messages. Tag questions make declarative statements less forceful: "It would mean a few hours of my time, *wouldn't it?"* Tag questions send a message of ambivalence and may imply that you are indecisive about what you intend to do.

Introductory disclaimers also make a statement less forceful and can contradict the intended meaning of the message. *"Don't get me wrong here*, but I think you should really take a good look at your relationship."

Other ambiguous types of messages include those that are posed as questions but are really statements of opinion, thought, or fact. "Don't you think the guest speaker was awful?" The question posed here is really a signal for a specific response and is a communication trap. Your opinion is not truly being solicited; what is sought is agreement with the opinion of another. Communicators can also give statements of their opinions posed as questions this way: "Are you *really* going to the dance dressed like that?"

Ambiguous messages may also carry a hidden agenda. For example, "Are you busy this weekend?" or "What are you doing tomorrow?" are questions with an agenda. Your friend may have plans for you. A clear way of stating this message would be, "I am moving this weekend/tomorrow. Are you available to help?"

CONVEYING MESSAGES THROUGH NONVERBAL BEHAVIOR

Actions speak louder than words. Nonverbal behavior conveys the intended meaning of a message without using words and helps communicators know how to interpret the message. You communicate nonverbally when you gesture, frown, smile, widen your eyes, move your chair closer to someone, raise your vocal volume, touch someone, or wear particular clothing.[5] It is not so much what we say but *how* we say it that helps others understand the meaning in messages. Verbal language conveys the content aspect of the message, such as statements of information, facts, thoughts, or feelings. Nonverbal behaviors communicate the relational aspect of the message, enabling communicators to convey how they feel about the subject they are discussing and how they feel about each other.

Albert Mehrabian's classic research findings indicate that as much as 93% of the total impact of a message is due to nonverbal behavior[6]:

- 38% of a message is conveyed through vocal tone and expression in voice
- 55% of a message is conveyed through facial expression and gestures
- Only 7% of a message is conveyed through verbal language
- The main reason that nonverbal behavior can convey greater impact to a message than words is that spoken words typically stimulate only the auditory sense of hearing, while nonverbal behaviors trigger several senses: visual, tactile, olfactory, and auditory. "People can understand nonverbal communication almost as a universal standard; it is an elaborate, secret code that is written nowhere yet understood by all."[7] Nonverbal communication behaviors serve many functions as shown in Table 4.1.[3,8]

TABLE 4.1	Functions of Nonverbal Communication Behaviors
Conveys emotions and feelings	Nonverbal communication is the richest source of information of your emotions and feelings.
Relatively free of deception	Nonverbal communication conveys intended meanings that are relatively free of deception. Words can conceal, deceive, and distort facts, thoughts, and feelings, whereas nonverbal communication is natural, automatic, and most often an unconscious act free of deception. However, people can convey false messages nonverbally, such as feigned interest in a subject or a fake smile.
Equivalent to a picture	Nonverbal communication is the equivalent of a "picture is worth a thousand words" during interpersonal, nurse-patient, and interdisciplinary communications.
Shorthand for words	Gestures such as "thumbs up," rolling your eyes, pointing to your watch, and a friendly wink are efficient ways of conveying a message.
Regulates conversation	Nonverbal communication can help regulate conversations with others. We often use hand signals to indicate "I am turning the table over to you" or lowering or raising the pitch in our voice to signal we are at the end of our conversation and that it is now someone else's turn.
Offers a safe way to express emotions	Nonverbal communication represents the most favorable means for expressing emotions indirectly. When you like someone, you may test the water first by flirting as opposed to verbally stating you like them. It is a means to save face and protect self-esteem.
Reinforces verbal message	Nonverbal behavior can reinforce a verbal message. You may say to someone to go north about two blocks and point in the appropriate direction.
Replaces words	Nonverbal behavior can replace words. Your classmate can turn to you and ask if you understood the instructions, and you may respond by shaking your head or shrugging your shoulders.
Provides emphasis	Nonverbal behavior can accentuate the verbal message by placing emphasis on certain words within a sentence through the tone in your voice.
Solves incongruence between verbal and nonverbal behavior	Nonverbal behavior prevails. When someone is visibly upset yet denies being upset when asked, assign more meaning to the nonverbal behavior than to the spoken words.

Communication Safety Alert

Nurses must carefully assess both the words and nonverbal behavior of patients. As a high-level communicator, always pay attention for any incongruence between the verbal and nonverbal message. If there is incongruence, believe the nonverbal behavior rather than the spoken words.

Nonverbal behaviors that are particularly important to be aware of in yourself and others include facial expressions, eye contact, paralanguage, gestures, clothing, proxemics, and touch. Nurses must effectively use nonverbal behaviors to establish and maintain nurse-patient and interdisciplinary relationships.

Facial expressions. The human face is the most expressive part of the human body. Research reveals that the human face is capable of producing over 250,000 types of expressions.[9,10] Facial expressions communicate emotional meaning more accurately than any other nonverbal behavior.[10] Through facial expressions, individuals provide nonverbal signals or clues that reveal their reactions to the verbal and nonverbal behaviors of others.

Eye contact. Eye contact can convey a great deal of information. We establish eye contact with another communicator because it is a classic signal (in Western culture) that we are interested in opening communications. We convey interest and that we are paying attention to the conversation by maintaining eye contact. We maintain eye contact to determine others' nonverbal reactions to our messages and to gauge if others are responding the way we had anticipated. When we look at the other communicators, we can gauge if they are having difficulty in understanding the intended meaning of our messages.

Tone of voice, also known as paralanguage. The human voice has many characteristics that can alter the way words are spoken. This is called paralanguage. Paralanguage is defined as the non-linguistic means of vocal expression; for example, tone, pitch, and volume.[8] Paralanguage conveys attitudes on a particular subject, mood, and feelings about others. By changing vocal rate, tone, pitch, and volume, we can give the same words different meanings.

Gestures. Body gestures convey attitudes and reinforce facial and paralanguage communication. Body gestures are also called body language. The way people nod their head, wave their hands, and position themselves reveals acceptance or bias about a certain topic or how much they like or dislike the communicator.[11]

Clothing. Clothing reveals emotions. When we are feeling depressed, we may feel most comfortable in loose clothing or pajamas. When feeling highly confident, we may feel like wearing our best outfit. The style of dress gives others cues on how to respond. Clothing can change our behavior and the behavior of others toward us. You behave differently when you are in your nursing uniform as opposed to when you are wearing jeans and a T-shirt. People will respond to you differently when you are wearing your nursing uniform than when you are wearing street clothing. Clothing conveys the following nonverbal messages to others:[12]

- Economic level
- Educational level
- Trustworthiness
- Social position

- Level of sophistication
- Social background
- Level of success
- Moral character

Proxemics: Proxemics refers to how people use space around them. Each of us maintains an invisible bubble, or *personal space,* that gives us psychological comfort when we interact with others. Hall[13] describes four comfort zones:

- *Intimate comfort zone:* In this zone, individuals are allowed into our most personal space. This typically reflects emotional closeness that involves skin contact, such as a hug from a parent, friend, spouse, or child, and represents a surrounding distance of 0 to 1.5 feet (0 to 0.5 meters).
- *Personal comfort zone:* This zone ranges from 1.5 to 4 feet (0.5 to 1.5 meters). This zone represents the space where most of our conversations with family, friends, and colleagues occur. When people we do not know well enter this zone, or when anyone comes into closer proximity to us than our personal preference, we may feel uncomfortable because our personal space has been invaded. Personal comfort zone is dependent on the culture of the individual. Women tend to stand in closer proximity to others than men.[14,15]
- *Social comfort zone:* Our comfort zone in social contexts is approximately 4 to 12 feet (1.5 to 3.5 meters). Group interactions typically occur within this space.
- *Public comfort zone:* This zone exceeds 12 feet (3.5 meters) Many public speakers and instructors position themselves within this zone.

Communication Safety Alert

Think of proxemics when you interact with patients. You enter their intimate and personal comfort zones each time you approach them to provide nursing care. Let patients know you plan to enter their personal comfort zone prior to touching them. You have to let patients know you plan to touch them by indirectly asking permission. For example, if you say "I need to check your blood pressure now," this is preparing patients prior to touching them. Before you enter a personal comfort zone, you need to warn the patient. In contrast, you would not just walk into a room and lift up the patient's gown to do an abdominal assessment without letting the patient know what you plan to do. This professional behavior promotes development of a trusting nurse-patient relationship.

Touch: Whether through a welcoming handshake with a friend or holding the patient's hand during an invasive procedure, the use of touch is a nonverbal expression of appreciation, acceptance, emotional support, encouragement, and praise when done appropriately. Because touch is also a behavior of sexual intimacy, there are legalities and social norms for interpersonal and professional touch behavior.

SENDING THE MESSAGE: CHOOSING THE APPROPRIATE CHANNEL OF COMMUNICATION

A key feature of high-level communication competency is choosing the channel that is the most appropriate to convey the intended meaning of the message. If you have had a heated conversation with someone and want to apologize, sending an e-mail is not appropriate.

Rather, meeting the individidual in person for a face-to-face discussion may be a better choice. When giving directions to someone who has never been to your house, it may be best to write them down or send them as a text message.

Once messages are conveyed through a channel, we need to understand the process of listening and then know how to respond effectively to what others say. Through purposeful listening and patient-safe listening responses, we can increase our ability to negotiate common meaning with others and interpret the meaning in messages as intended.

RECEIVING AND RESPONDING TO MESSAGES: LISTENING

Approximately 70% of communication activity is spent on listening.[16] Despite the importance of listening, most people are not effective listeners.

The Listening Process

Listening, as opposed to simply hearing, is the way we make sense out of what we hear. It is a complex process that involves five components:[1]

- **Hearing:** The first electrophysiological trigger for the listening event.
- **Attending:** Selecting the stimuli through our perceptual filter.
- **Understanding:** Interpreting the stimuli by assigning meaning.
- **Remembering:** Transferring the meaning into memory for later recall.
- **Responding:** Confirm that listening has occurred by providing verbal and nonverbal feedback by using listening responses.

Hearing is only the first stage of the listening process. The listening process is interactive because it includes providing feedback to the speaker through listening responses that convey our understanding of the message. The listening responses are verbal and nonverbal messages sent to the other communicator. Through listening responses, interpretations of messages can be clarified and verified to achieve the highest probability that messages are understood as intended.

High-level communicators understand that listening responses are vital to creating common meaning and shared understanding between communicators. The way individuals respond to messages with feedback reveals if they are really listening and processing what is said and how they are interpreting messages. Effective listening responses provide the necessary feedback to the speaker that indicate if the message is understood as intended or if the message needs to be corrected and clarified to ensure the creation of common meaning.

The most accurately stated message delivered through a carefully selected channel will not be effective if the receiver does not respond with feedback using effective listening responses. Because the listening process involves interpretation and feedback to confirm the meaning of the message, listening responsively is often referred to as "active" listening.

There are several risk factors that create interference and block the ability to listen and respond effectively to messages, thereby hindering creation of common meaning between communicators. These factors must be recognized and overcome, as they can lead to communication breakdowns, miscommunications, and frustration in personal and professional relationships.

Listening Risk Factors

Factors that pose risk to listening effectively are those that interfere with our ability to hear and to interpret, and those that distract the focus of our attention from the message that we are receiving. These include internal physiological factors, information overload, brain processing, and external physical factors. [1,8]

- Internal **Physiological factors:** Internal factors, such as hearing impairment, cognitive impairment, anxiety, nervousness, fatigue, pain, sedation, and feeling stressed or ecstatic, interfere with listening to others with accuracy.
- **Overload:** If a person is in information overload, they simply cannot process other information. Individuals tune out communication stimuli. The health-care setting is complex with patient details to remember, protocols to implement, medications to administer and record, and patients that leave and return to the unit. Given all these events, people sometimes cannot absorb yet more data.
- **Brain processing:** The mind can process messages of up to 600 words per minute,[17] whereas the average person speaks approximately 100 to 140 words per minute. As a consequence, people may plan what to say next while the other person is still talking or let their attention wander. Communication breakdown occurs when communicators are not fully focused on creating common meaning of the intended message.
- **Physical noise:** External factors, such as physical distractions, unfamiliar sounds, and sounds that call attention away from the conversation, interfere with accurate listening. The setting of the communication situation can interfere with listening, such as communicating on the phone while others are in conversation close by. The health-care setting is noisy with many distractions and interruptions that can lead to communication breakdown.

In addition, there are blocking verbal responses to messages that lead to communication breakdowns. Communicators need to know what *not* to say when providing feedback to a message.

Blocking the Expression of Thoughts and Feelings

We may be tempted to come to the emotional rescue of others because of our own discomfort in certain communication situations.[18] We try to prevent the other person from reacting emotionally to the situation. Although this may seem well-intended, this is a detrimental and misguided approach to communicating because we are not allowing the other person to express thoughts and feelings. These are blocking responses that are to be avoided because they shut down communication. When patients are blocked from expression of emotions and feelings by health-care providers, they lose trust in them and do not share information. This can lead to unsafe situations.

Claiming another's feelings as your own: Statements such as "I know how you must be feeling" claim another's feelings. This makes people angry because it belittles feelings that are unique to them. They typically respond, "You have no idea how I am feeling. How could you know? You are not me."

Denying others the right to their feelings: Comments such as, "Don't worry about it," "It could happen to anyone," or "You'll get over it," deny and invalidate the feelings of others. Doing so cuts off continued communication by making communicators feel anxious because they perceive there is something wrong with how they uniquely feel.

Showing disapproval: Statements such as "Why are you getting so angry? There's no reason for it" express disapproval. These statements belittle people's feelings and may yield shame. You do not have to agree with others; rather, convey a willingness to listen to another's viewpoint, then agree to disagree on the topic.

Challenging statements: When you ask an individual a question that begins with "why," you are attacking the person and putting him or her on the defensive. Consider this question, "Why are you not taking your medications?" This sounds accusatory and laden with your judgment that the patient has done something wrong. Rather, ask the question this way, "I see that you are not taking your medications. Could you tell me more about this?" Try to ask questions that begin with "who," "what," "where," "when," and "how" instead of "why."

Giving false reassurance: This includes comments such as, "It is probably nothing" or "I am sure the tests will show nothing abnormal." These clichés are attempts to pretend everything is fine and to cover up emotions. False reassurance denies individuals the ability to express their emotions and concerns and can violate the trust between nurse and patient.

Minimizing the situation: Similar to false reassurance, minimizing includes responses such as, "It's just some blood tests" or "It's not so bad." These responses deny the individual the right to express concerns and fears and invalidate the extent of the emotions the individual may be feeling.

Imposing guilt: Do not make people feel guilty about their emotions, concerns, and fears. Imagine a nurse responding to a crying patient by saying, "You need to compose yourself. You know how important it is to be strong. Think of your family." The patient was feeling vulnerable; now the patient is also feeling guilt.

Giving advice: Giving advice proclaims your lack of faith in the ability of others to think for themselves and make their own decisions. You imply you are the only one who knows what is best. Giving advice denies individuals the ability to become self-directing agents in managing issues, problem solving, and coping.

Reacting with defensiveness: Responding defensively means you are taking something personally. Your response may sound like an attack on another. For example, the patient states, "One of the staff members stole my purse." You respond, "I highly doubt anyone in this hospital would steal your purse." You are being both defensive and confrontational.

    In both your personal and professional life, it is important to avoid feedback that blocks communication. The next section of the chapter focuses on patient-safe communication strategies that are active and effective listening responses that facilitate high-level communication.

Patient-Safe Communication Strategies

Patient-safe communication strategies that represent effective listening responses are termed "active" or "facilitative" because patients are encouraged to express thoughts and feelings. These responses promote the development of trust in professional relationships. Active listening responses ensure the creation of common meaning and understanding between communicators. Specific patient-safe verbal responses are used to clarify and verify messages. By clarifying and validating our interpretation of a message, we have the highest probability of creating common meaning between ourselves and others. Nurses pay careful attention to patients who are speaking and use deliberate critical thought processing to make sense of a message. Nurses then validate the intended meaning of the message through active listening responses that provide feedback to patients that they understand the intended message.

Paraphrasing

Paraphrasing is feedback that restates, in your own words, the message you thought a communicator sent. The following narrative shows the effects of paraphrasing in the communication situation:

> PATIENT: "I am really tired of all the blood they are taking from me. They are poking me every 4 hours.

> PARAPHRASING RESPONSE: "It sounds like you are frustrated with all of these blood tests and this is hurting you."

> Paraphrasing draws out more information from the individual and can add a deeper understanding of what the underlying issues really are:

> PATIENT: "Well, you are sort of right, I guess. I want to go home so I can be with my family, not be here and constantly pinched and prodded. It's making me angry."

Listening With Silence

Through purposeful active listening with silence, we can show our concern and support by giving people uninterrupted time to collect their thoughts and consider how they want to express their thoughts. Even through silence, we are communicating a response to a message.

Questioning

Listeners respond by questioning when they need additional information to understand the message. This includes closed-ended and open-ended questions. Closed-ended questions require a factual response that is answered with a yes, no, or maybe. For example, "Would you say that your breathing has improved following your ventolin treatment?" In contrast, open-ended questions facilitate verbal and nonverbal explanation of facts, thoughts, and feelings. Such questions cannot be answered with a yes or no. For example, "How was your ventolin treatment?" is open-ended, requiring the expression of thoughts about the treatment.

Empathy

Empathy is defined as the ability to experience the feelings of another individual from that individual's own unique perspective.[8] It provides an understanding that is more than verbal acknowledgement of the feelings of another. It is an opportunity to "step into someone else's shoes" for a time to experience the emotions of another. There are significant positive outcomes of using empathy during interpersonal communications. For the person receiving empathy, there is an increase in self-esteem by knowing that the other communicator is actively listening and is willing to accept personal thoughts and feelings without any evaluations or judgments. The person feels not only heard but understood, and a deeper sense of trust develops.

Patients express clues subtly about their desire to discuss their emotions during interactions with health-care providers. A study by Levinson, Gorawara-Bhat, and

Lamb[19] demonstrated that when physicians missed opportunities to offer an empathetic response, patients offered clues repeatedly. When their needs for having their feelings acknowledged empathetically were not met, patients searched for a new physician. Studies reveal that empathetic communication improves patient health outcomes,[20] increases compliance with treatment,[21] and increases provider and patient satisfaction.[22,23] To offer empathy effectively:

1. Recognize the presence of a patient's strong feelings in the clinical setting (i.e., fear, anger, grief, disappointment)
2. Imagine how the patient might be feeling
3. State your perception of the patient's feeling (i.e., "I can imagine that must be...." or "It sounds like you're upset about....")
4. Legitimize the feeling: "It's alright to feel angry right now...."
5. Respect the patient's effort to cope with the predicament
6. Offer support and partnership (i.e., "I'm committed to work with you to...." or "Let's see what we can do together to....")

Summarizing
Summarizing provides the opportunity to review and validate the major points within the communication situation. For example, it can be used as a patient-safe strategy when providing patient education. "Today, we reviewed what you can expect before, during, and after surgery. Is there anything we missed or anything else you would like to talk about?"

Supportive Statements
Supportive statements include an agreement with the communicator's perspective: "I think you are on the right track here." In addition, supportive statements include offering to help, such as, "I am here if you need to talk."

Analytical Statements
Responding with an analytical statement means you offer an interpretation of the individual's message. The goal of using analytical statements is to help individuals see a situation within a broader perspective and with greater objectivity. An analytical statement may be transformational and help individuals consider meanings in situations they may not have thought of from their own perspective. "I think what you are really saying is...." or "Maybe what is really going on is...."

Evaluative Statements
Evaluative statements are used to offer encouragement as well as constructive feedback, such as "Look how well you are walking today—good for you!" Evaluative statements that provide constructive feedback can promote patient safety. "Everything looked good when you were drawing up your own insulin. I just got the sense that we may need to work on your understanding of why you draw up short-acting insulin first. Let's try it again and have you talk through it as if you were teaching me." Always start constructive feedback with a positive statement, and then introduce an objective observation of behavior that reveals an opportunity for improvement.

Which Patient-Safe Active Listening Response Should You Use?
Research shows that each of the listening responses has the potential to contribute to negotiating common meaning and enhancing the relationship within which the meaning

exists.[24] There are several factors to take into consideration when selecting an appropriate response:

- Think about the context of the situation. At times it is best to be encouraging and supportive; at other times you may need to offer an analysis of the situation.
- Think about individual people. Can they come to their own solutions through paraphrasing and open questioning, or do they need more analytical responses? Can they accept constructive feedback?
- Think about your own comfort and skill when making selections.
- In nursing, you will need to develop skill in each of the patient-safe active listening responses to negotiate meaning effectively, appropriately, and sensitively within a wide range of patient situations.

CHAPTER SUMMARY

This chapter focused on sending, receiving, and responding to messages to attain the highest level of probability in achieving common meaning and shared understanding between communicators. Specifically, the chapter described how communicators use verbal language and nonverbal behaviors to convey messages and choose a specific channel and how they use the listening process to interpret and validate the intended meaning of messages through patient-safe active listening responses. Nurses must overcome factors that pose risk to listening, such as physiological factors, information overload, brain processing, and physical noise, through patient-safe facilitative active listening responses.

BUILDING HIGH-LEVEL COMMUNICATION COMPETENCE

For additional exercises, visit DavisPlus at http://davisplus.fadavis.com

1. **Reflective Practice.** Reflective practice is a self-regulating, active process of stepping back and witnessing one's own experience, then examining the experience in greater depth. Think about and write a one-page summary of a recent communication situation that did not go as you had planned. Explain the verbal language used in the message, the means to convey the message, and listening responses. Specify what you will do differently the next time a similar situation occurs.

2. **Communication Practice.** Work with a classmate to complete the following activities:

   a. Sit with your backs to each other. Tell your partner how to get from your education institution to your home using the communication process and listening responses to negotiate mutual understanding. As you provide the directions, your partner will draw a map. At the end of the exercise, look at the map, and determine its accuracy.

   b. Are you aware of your personal comfort zone? Work with your partner to determine your personal space. How close do you usually stand to someone when you converse with him or her?

   c. Communicate a story to your partner using nonverbal behavior only.

3. **Critical Thinking**

   a. Paraphrase the following statement, "You make me so mad when you leave the bathroom a mess."

   b. A patient states the following during the health history, "My asthma is getting the best of me and my enjoyment of life. I really feel that I am missing so much in life." You recognize the strong feelings of the patient. What type of response would be prudent in this situation?

4. **Critical Thinking.** What are the words and nonverbal behaviors a nurse may use to obtain personal health information from patients? Why is it important that nurses negotiate common meaning with patients?

References

1. Beebe, S.A., Beebe, S.J., Redmond, M.V., et al. Interpersonal Communication, 4th ed. Toronto, Ontario, Pearson Education Canada: 2007.
2. Griffin, K., Patton, B.R. Fundamentals of Interpersonal Communication, 2nd ed. N.Y., Harper & Row: 1976.
3. Weaver, R.L. Understanding Interpersonal Communication. 7th ed. N.Y., Addison-Wesley: 1996.
4. Levinson, S.C. Pragmatics. Cambridge, England, Cambridge University: 1983.
5. DeVito, J.A. The Interpersonal Communication Book, 11th ed. Boston, Pearson Education, Allyn and Bacon: 2007.
6. Mehrabian, A. Silent Messages: Implicit Communication of Emotions and Attitudes, 2nd ed. Belmont, Calif., Wadsworth Publishing: 1981.

7. Sapir, E., The Unconscious Patterning of Behavior in Society. In Mandelbaum, D., ed. Selected Writings of Edward Sapir in Language, Culture, and Personality. Berkeley, Calif., University of California Press: 1949, p. 556.

8. Adler, R.B., Rosenfeld, L.B., Proctor, R.F., et al. Interplay: The Process of Interpersonal Communication. Don Mills, Ontario, Oxford University Press: 2006.

9. Ekman, P., Friesen, W.V., Tomkins, S.S. Facial Affect Scoring Technique (FAST): A First Validity Study. Semiotica 3:37-38, 1971.

10. Ekman, P., Friesen, W.V. Unmasking the Face. A Guide to Recognizing Emotions From Facial Clues. Englewood Cliffs, N.J., Prentice-Hall: 1975.

11. Mehrabian, A. Nonverbal Communication. Chicago, Aldine-Atherton: 1972.

12. Thourlby, W. You Are What You Wear. N.Y., New American Library: 1978.

13. Hall, E.T. The Hidden Dimension. Garden City, N.Y., Anchor: 1969.

14. Sommer, R. Studies in Personal Space. Sociometry 22:247-260, 1959.

15. Knapp, M.L., Hall, J.A. Nonverbal Communication in Human Interaction, 3rd ed, Fort Worth Tex., Holt, Rinehart and Winston: 1992.

16. Steil, L.K. Listening Training: The Key to Success in Today's Organizations. In Purdy, M., Borisoff, D., eds. Listening in Everyday life: A Personal and Professional Approach, 2nd ed. Lanham Md., University Press of America: 1996, pp. 213-237.

17. Versfeld, N.J., Dreschler, W.A. The Relationship Between the Intelligibility of Time-Compressed Speech and Speech-In-Noise in Young and Elderly Listeners. Journal of the Acoustical Society of America 111:401-408, 2002.

18. Iveson-Iveson, J. The Art of Communication. Nursing Mirror 156:47, 1983.

19. Levinson, W., Gorawara-Bhat, R., Lamb, J. A Study of Patient Clues and Physician Responses in Primary Care and Surgical Settings. Journal of the American Medical Association 284:1021-1027, 2000.

20. Stewart, MA. Effective Physician-Patient Communication and Health Outcomes: A Review. Canadian Medical Association Journal 152:1423-1433, 1995.

21. Stewart, MA. What Is a Successful Doctor-Patient Interview? A Study of Interactions and Outcomes. Social Science and Medicine 19:167-175, 1984.

22. Suchman, A.L., Roter, D., Green, M., et al.: Physician Satisfaction With Primary Care Office Visits. Collaborative Study Group of the American Academy on Physicians and Patients. Medical Care 31:1083-1092, 1993.

23. Brody, D.S., Miller, S.M., Lerman, C.E., et al.: The Relationship Between Patients' Satisfaction With Their Physicians and Perceptions About Interventions They Desired and Received. Medical Care 27:1027-1035, 1989.

24. Burleson, B.R. Comforting Messages: Features, Functions and Outcomes. In Daly, J.A., Wienmann, J.M., eds. Strategic Interpersonal Communication. Hillsdale, N.J., Lawrence Erlbaum: 1994, pp. 135-161.

Culture and Gender Issues in Patient-Safe Communication

Upon completion of this chapter, you will be able to:

1. Describe the importance of the contexts of culture and gender within the transformational model of communication.
2. Explain how personal cultural values and beliefs can interfere with negotiation and creation of common meaning.
3. Identify the importance of understanding gender and cultural differences in patient-safe communication.
4. Give examples of gender differences in communication that can interfere with negotiation and creation of common meaning.
5. Identify patient-safe communication strategies to build cross-cultural and gender-specific high-level communication competency.

Key Words

Culture
Gender
Ethnicity

Cultural value
Cultural belief
Spirituality

In this chapter, you will learn the importance of assessing the patient's cultural beliefs and practices and gender differences in communication. Both will affect the patient-safe strategies needed to devise, implement, and evaluate plans of care for patients in health-care settings. This chapter expands upon the context ring of the Transformational Model of Communication and the importance of recognizing and working within appropriate contexts to have the best chance of successful transformational outcomes in health care. Review the context ring of the Transformational Model of Communication in Chapter 2.

Health-care providers must be resourceful and creative to tailor interventions to suit the patient's culture.[1] They must respect differences and appreciate the inherent worth of diverse cultures.[2] Patient-safe, culturally competent communication is required in order to have the best chance of negotiating common meaning for all aspects of patient care management.

The first step in becoming a patient-safe, culturally competent nurse is to become aware of, and reflect upon, your own values, attitudes, and beliefs. The second step is to assess the patient's cultural values, attitudes, and beliefs. You analyze how they are alike or different from your own in order to develop your awareness and increase your cultural sensitivity. The more culturally sensitive you become, the better able you will be to negotiate common meaning with your patients and prevent miscommunications that may lead to harmful events. *For an interactive version of this activity, see DavisPlus at http://davisplus.fadavis.com*

You may be surprised to learn that the 20 value statements listed online have been derived from the culture of North Americans. L. Robert Kohls,[3] past Executive Director of The Washington International Center and current Director of International Programs at San Francisco State University, has developed a guide intended to explain to a foreigner the verbal and nonverbal behaviors of Americans, "actions which might otherwise appear to be strange, confusing, or unbelievable, when evaluated from the perspective of the foreigner's own society and its values."[3] We need to take a look at ourselves from the perspective of "foreigners," so that we can get to know who we are and how our own values have a direct impact on our communications and the safe and effective delivery of patient care.

PERSONAL CONTROL OVER THE ENVIRONMENT

North Americans typically believe that people should control nature and everything in their environments that affects them. North Americans feel compelled to do (one way or another) what the majority of the world is certain cannot be done.[3] For example, stem cell research and genetic engineering are being conducted to control every disease and grow back amputated limbs.

If patients hold more traditional values, they may believe that bad luck and fate are responsible for their problems in life and that many things are out of their control. Nurses spend time teaching patients how to control their illnesses and need to take into consideration the patients' views on what they believe they can and cannot control.

Change

In North America, change is seen as good and is linked to progress and growth.[3] In contrast, patients with traditional values who want to hold onto traditions consider change to be disruptive and destructive and will avoid change in favor of stability, continuity, and heritage. With many illnesses, behavioral change is needed, and this creates conflict for many individuals who do not want to change their lifestyles.

Time and Its Control

In North America, time is of critical importance, and things must be accomplished according to predetermined schedules. It is considered rude to be late for an appointment, and an individual should always phone if unavoidably detained. To patients from traditional cultures, North Americans may be viewed as being more interested in getting things done on time than in developing and maintaining interpersonal relationships.[3] In nursing, it is important to get patient care activities done on time *and* to maintain interpersonal relationships with your patients.

Equality

For North Americans, there is a belief that all people are "created equal," which reflects a religious basis, that God views all humans alike without regard to intelligence, physical characteristics, or economic status. In those from traditional cultures, rank, status, and authority are more desirable to promote a sense of order, security, and certainty. They find it reassuring to know who they are and where they fit into society.[3] Patients from traditional backgrounds may treat physicians and nurses with deferential manners and high respect, because they view them as authority figures. Traditional views may inhibit patients from viewing themselves as integral parts of the health-care team.

Individualism and Privacy

Individuals in North America believe themselves to be unique, totally different from everyone else, and resist thinking of themselves as part of any homogeneous group. There is emphasis on individuality, not on belonging to groups as in traditional cultures. Traditional cultures focus on the needs of the group, not on the needs of individuals.[3]

Stemming from the value of individualism is a belief in privacy, seen in such statements as, "If I don't have at least half an hour to myself a day, I will go stark raving mad." The word "privacy" does not even exist in many cultures, or it has a negative connotation of loneliness.[3]

North American health care emphasizes the uniqueness of individuals and protects the privacy of patients through the confidentiality of health-related information. In patients from traditional cultures with an emphasis on the group, there may be many family members in the waiting room, and they may all be asking for confidential information about their family members. Nurses, who are focused on the needs of the patient and the family group, must protect the privacy of the patient and maintain positive family relationships. Family group members may want to be actively involved in the care of one of their group members and want to feed or bathe the patient or perform other care-related activities. Nurses may enlist the help of family members in the care of patients when family members want to participate in the care of one of their "group." Nurses also need to explain privacy laws and regulations to family members so that they understand the principles of confidentiality.

Self-Help

Closely related to individualism is the idea of self-help. In the English language, there are more than 100 words about doing things for one's self,[3] These words include self-confidence, self-conscious, self-contented, self-control, self-discipline, self-expression, and so on. Most other languages do not contain the equivalent words containing "self."[3] In nursing, there is emphasis placed on "self-care." Nurses may assume that all patients want to perform their own care so that they can regain their independence. Those with traditional values may be perfectly content to have others make decisions and manage their care.

Competition and Free Enterprise

The belief that competition "brings out the best in everyone" is a North American ideal.[3] The economic system of free enterprise is also based on the idea that because competition brings out the best in people, society will progress rapidly. In North America, health-care systems compete for patients and government funding; health-care workers compete for promotions; and patients compete for services provided by health-care organizations. Patients from traditional cultures may find competition disagreeable when they value cooperation and cohesiveness to avoid conflict and jealousy among group members.[3]

Future Orientation

North Americans value the future and the improvements the future will bring.[3] They devalue the past and do not dwell on past events.[3] Even a happy present time may go largely unnoticed because North Americans are hopeful the future will bring even greater happiness. In some patients from traditional cultures, talking about or planning the future is felt to be futile if they believe fate controls their destiny and there is nothing that can be done. Traditional cultures live for the present and value the past.[3]

Viewed through the values of North American health-care providers, past orientation and belief in fate can make traditional patients appear to be superstitious, lazy, and unwilling to take the initiative to bring about improvements. Instead, if nurses recognize the past orientation, they need to focus on planning with patients by "taking one day at a time."

Action and Work Orientation

North Americans routinely plan an extremely active day and believe in the "dignity" of human labor.[3] It is believed to be "sinful" to waste one's time. North Americans believe leisure activities should occupy a small portion of time during one's life and should be used to refresh one's energy so that one has the ability to work harder and more productively upon return to work.[3]

In contrast, there is a "being" orientation in some cultures and a focus on living in the present.[3] When a patient says, "I want to be left alone to talk on the phone and sleep today," and the health-care system operates on the North American cultural value of "Don't just lie there; you need to do something to make yourself better," conflicts are going to arise. Nurses realize patients have the right to refuse treatments and medications, yet have often wondered, "Why is he refusing to cooperate?" or "What is he thinking?" The answer to these questions may lie in different cultural orientations to action.

Informality

North Americans are very informal and casual.[3] For example, bosses urge their employees to call them by their first names and feel uncomfortable being called "Mr." or "Mrs." To those of other cultures, this informality may be unsettling and considered disrespectful and insulting.[3] Nurses need to find out how their patients prefer to be addressed, and let patients decide how they want to address nurses. Patients may feel more comfortable calling their nurse Mr. or Mrs. instead of by a first name. In addition, it is very important that nurses present a professional image through professional dress and manners, further described in Unit 2.

Directness, Openness, and Honesty

North Americans are likely to deliver negative evaluations or unpleasant information honestly and directly and may be very blunt. North Americans value assertiveness and a direct and open approach.[3] In contrast, patients from other cultures may have developed subtle ways of informing people of unpleasant news or negative evaluations.[3] Directness, openness, and especially bluntness can be very shocking and disturbing to patients who do not value a direct approach to receiving unpleasant information.

Health-care providers sometimes relay bad news and must learn high-level communication strategies to deliver bad news in a gentle manner. Not all people appreciate the blunt "give me the news straight" approach and need to be eased into the bad news. Nurses need to use active listening and offer emotionally supportive responses when patients and families receive bad news.

Practicality and Efficiency

North Americans value practicality and efficiency and devalue emotions and sentimentality.[3] Practical considerations are given the highest priority before making a decision. Examples of this value include: "Will it pay its own way?," "What can be gained from the activity?," "Will it make any money?" Problem solving involves listing several solutions and then trying them out, one by one, to see which works best.

Other cultures do not place such emphasis on pragmatism and may focus on idealism.[3] For example, the emphasis is on aesthetics and beauty instead of practicality and efficiency. In North American health-care situations, sentimentality and emotions do not take precedence over the practical aspects of patient care. Many patients are very emotional, especially about health-care problems and the stress associated with illness. Nurses must learn to give emotionally supportive responses to patients. Although health-care providers may be able to be quite objective and rational about the patients' situation, they need to be able to see beyond the practical and be sensitive to emotions of patients and families who feel overwhelmed with the situation.

Materialism and Acquisitiveness

North Americans consider material objects a natural benefit of hard work that all people could enjoy if they were as industrious and hard-working.[3] North Americans place a higher priority on obtaining, maintaining, and protecting their material objects than in developing and enjoying interpersonal relationships.[3] These views are very different from cultural values that emphasize spiritualism. Spirituality is about religious beliefs and includes behaviors that provide meaning in life. The emphasis is placed on developing relationships with a higher power and meaningful interpersonal relationships on earth. Spirituality is reflected, for example, in the belief that we are put here on earth to help one another, not to see who can accumulate the most material possessions.[3] During times of sickness, many patients question their spirituality, and nurses need to explore what gives meaning to the life of their patients and identify the sources of inner strength to help patients cope with their problems.

CULTURAL ASSESSMENT

The only way to deliver culturally competent care is by using high-level communication competency to assess culture and determine the impact of the recommended plan of treatment on the values and beliefs of the patient and family. Box 5.1 is a cultural assessment used in health-care settings based on the work of Purnell and Paulanka.[4,5]

BOX 5.1 *Cultural Assessment*

- **Heritage:** What is the patient's country of origin? Is the patient familiar with the health-care system and health-care providers in this country?
- **Communication:** Are there language barriers? Will the patient feel comfortable sharing his thoughts and feelings?
- **Family Roles and Organization:** Who is the dominant member of the household, the person in the family who is the spokesperson and decision maker?
- **Biocultural Ecology:** What are the specific genetic or environmentally transmitted diseases that cause health problems in the different cultural groups?
- **High-Risk Behaviors:** Does the cultural group use tobacco, alcohol, or recreational drugs? Is participation in high-risk physical activities common? Is there a lack of adherence to important health safety practices?
- **Nutrition:** What are the basic ingredients of native food dishes and preparation practices?
- **Pregnancy and Childbearing Practices:** What are the preferences for birth control methods, the roles of men in childbirth, the positions for delivering a baby, and the preferred types of health practitioners (male or female, midwife or obstetrician)?
- **Death Rituals:** What is the patient's view of death, dying, and the afterlife?
- **Spirituality:** What is the patient's dominant religion and views regarding the meaning and purpose of life?
- **Health-Seeking Beliefs and Behaviors:** What are the patient's beliefs about pain, mental and physical handicaps, chronic illness, and folklore practices?

Communication Safety Alert

It is impossible to know the beliefs and practices of every culture, but health-care providers who are intent on providing patient-safe, culturally competent care continue to learn by assessing their patient's culture, traveling, reading, and attending events held by local ethnic and cultural organizations.

GENDER

It is necessary to understand the impact of gender in interpersonal relationships and health care.[6] Gender differences in communication are partially derived from cultural backgrounds. The purpose of recognizing gender differences in styles of communication is to understand ourselves and members of the opposite sex, and to apply this knowledge to facilitate communication between men and women and to increase the probability of negotiating and creating common meaning. You must be able to assess each person's gender-specific verbal and nonverbal communications and then adjust your communication to have the highest probability of negotiating and creating common meaning with patients and other health-care providers.

Cultural Influences on Gender Communications

Communication between genders has been called cross-cultural communication; it reflects the different beliefs and practices of men and women affecting interpersonal relationships. Verbal and nonverbal behavior of men and women involve cultural gender-specific ideas and practices that have been learned through socialization with family and other significant groups.

Gender Roles

Gender roles consist of the different activities that men and women engage in with different frequencies.[7] The roles of women and men are culturally encouraged patterns of behavior. Thus, verbal and nonverbal behaviors for communication are part of gender role.

Gender roles have changed over time because of the changing needs of society. Ideas about acceptable gender-specific behaviors in others and ourselves are constantly under revision. For example, women are expected to be gentle and emotional; men are expected to be powerful and in control of their feelings. In recognizing these gender role differences, you are not stereotyping. Instead, you are classifying and identifying typical behavior patterns pertinent to communication based on gender.

Communication Safety Alert

Once you recognize typical gender differences in communication, you can modify your verbal and nonverbal behaviors to communicate messages with precision and clarity to members of the opposite sex.

In addition to cultural differences in gender communications, there are also biological influences.

Biological Influences

Although brain research is still in its infancy, neurologists suggest that there are structural and chemical differences in the brains of men and women.[7-9] Biological theories suggest these differences influence human verbal and nonverbal behavior.

Research indicates that female brains are less lateralized during speech. Women use both sides of the brain, whereas men use primarily the left side of the brain, regardless of whether they are right-handed or left-handed.[9] In addition, men's brains are influenced by the hormone testosterone, whereas women's brains are primarily influenced by the hormones oxytocin, estrogen, and progesterone.[7,8,10,11] These hormones influence sexual development and verbal and nonverbal behavior.

For example, male bodies produce 10 to 40 times more testosterone than do female bodies.[10] Research suggests that aggressive behaviors may be linked to hormonal abnormalities and that men with higher-than-average testosterone levels exhibit a wide variety of antisocial behaviors.[7]

It will take many more years to sort out the biological and cultural differences in communication. In the meantime, researchers agree that men and women have different verbal and nonverbal styles of speech.[7,12-17] Your personal experiences communicating with members of the opposite sex may have already led you to the conclusion that differences do exist in communication patterns, although you may not have recognized and classified them.

Differences in Styles of Speech

Tannen's research identified several differences in the verbal and nonverbal styles of speech between men and women (primarily North American).[12,13] She compares and contrasts gender differences that may become communication barriers that are risk factors for clear communication between the sexes.

Tannen's research suggests that the communication style of women typically focuses on closeness and support to preserve intimacy in relationships and that men are focused on status and maintaining their independence. These are polar opposite views of the world and often result in conflict. For example, a man gets a call at work from an old friend who says he is in town for the weekend, and the man invites the friend to stay at his home. His wife is upset because he did not ask her first. He is angry because his status has been lowered, and his independence has been threatened if he has to tell his friend he cannot stay for the weekend. She is angry because he has not sought her consent whether the friend could stay for the weekend. Both husband and wife may end up in a battle thinking each other selfish.

Rapport Talk Versus Report Talk

Tannen suggests that communication tends to be unbalanced because men and women talk to accomplish different purposes.[12,13] For most women, the preferred language of everyday conversation is that of rapport. Women are interested in establishing and negotiating intimate, sympathetic, harmonious relationships. The essence of female friendship is to get together to talk about what they think and feel about a situation, with careful attention to details of what happened and who was there. As a result, many women can express what they are feeling better than many men can.

Communication Safety Alert

Rapport talk needs to be distinguished from destructive gossip, however. The difference between rapport talk, often characteristic of women, and gossip, is that gossip is destructive and involves rumors, slander, and defamation of character. Gossip does not create rapport between individuals.

If you realize, in health-care situations, that many women make small talk to establish rapport, even if you personally prefer a more direct or technical approach to a conversation, you become better able to understand the purpose of the other person's conversational style. In addition, it is interesting to note that in terms of total talking time observed in conversations, men spend more time talking than women.[14,15]

Report talk is characteristic of male language.[12,13] Men generally prefer a style of language that involves freely announcing and stating facts to give an account, with a "skip-the-details" approach.[12,13] In contrast to the speech style of many women, the purpose of the report style of speech for many men is to assert independence and to maintain or increase status in social groups.[12,13]

RAPPORT AND REPORTING SKILLS FOR NURSES

Regardless of the health-care setting in which you work, you will spend much of your time talking to patients and family members, other nurses, and other members of the health-care team. Rapport talk with patients is essential to patient-safe communication because it leads to the development of trusting nurse-patient relationships. Nurses typically take a patient-centered approach focused on interpersonal relationships with patients and their significant others.[18] Nurses also tend to focus on developing sympathetic and harmonious relationships. To care for patients successfully, you will need to assess carefully their physical and emotional responses and their adjustment to the hospital, clinic, or home care setting. You will learn the most intimate details of patients' health status and family situation, and then apply your knowledge as a health professional to provide physical and emotional support, guidance, and teaching.

You also need to know how to report information with a "skip-the-details" approach. For example, when you give an end-of-shift report to other nurses, you will want to provide only critical information. In talking with physicians about patients, report talk is definitely indicated. Physicians focus on the pathophysiology and are interested in a brief summary of the patient's physiological status. Tell the physician about vital signs and head-to-toe assessment data specific to the patient's malfunctioning physiological systems.

Less Adversative Versus More Adversative

The word *adversative* is defined as pitting one's own needs, wants, and skills against those of others.[12,13] In this context, it involves conflict, and it is an essential part of human nature. The way you learn to manage conflict may be related to the types of games you played as a child. Janet Lever studied fifth graders at play.[19] Boys' games involved complex rules and roles and relied on skills. In contrast, girls' games involved complexity in verbally managing interpersonal relations. Girls' games were contests but not of skill. Rather, games became a popularity contest. Lever suggested that the social games children play as they grow up contribute to the formation of adult responses to conflict.

To many women, conflict is a threat to connection and should be avoided.[12,13] The goal of conversation for many women is to strive for peace and harmony.[12,13] When it comes to a career and the workplace, women often place higher value on affiliation and collective goals than on personal achievement.[12,13] Women are inclined to sacrifice personal needs for the needs of the group. When it comes to making decisions, women tend to take into account more factors, with a higher sensitivity to personal and moral aspects of a problem.[12,13]

Many men are much more comfortable with competition and conflict. If the conflict is friendly, it becomes a means of bonding, for example in football or other sports. The perspective of many men is that some people are higher and some are lower in status in a social group. Everyone has a function, but not everyone is equal. If it comes to a choice between being liked or respected, many men would probably prefer to be respected.[12,13]

🧩 NURSES AND ADVERSITY

As a nurse, whether you are male or female, you must learn to manage conflict. You may encounter conflicts over scheduling or patient assignments, appropriate treatment measures, ethical issues, and other differences, regardless of the setting in which you work. If you have trouble dealing with adversity and conflict, you will need to come to terms with that problem. Although diplomacy and tact are essential skills, too much politeness may dilute the message.

You also must develop sensitivity to the moral and social aspects of patient care situations by learning to become a patient advocate. Advocacy in nursing means that you must speak up to defend human rights—the right of patients to make their own decisions, for example.

Cooperative Overlapping Versus Talking Alone

In a communication pattern known as overlapping, a listener may talk along with the speaker, yet the speaker is not annoyed or disturbed by the intrusion. The purpose of the overlap is to show support, interest, cooperation, and emotional ties. In contrast, an interruption is considered to be a violation of speaking rights and, thus, to be inconsiderate.[12,13]

Most North Americans believe that one person should speak at a time, although North American women overlap more than men do in an attempt to build relationships.[12,13] In many cases, North American men may consider the overlap an interruption, especially if they prefer to hold center stage as a means to demonstrate independence and status.[12,13]

The key to whether overlap becomes an interruption depends on whether the conversation is balanced. If both speakers cooperatively overlap each other, there is balance and harmony.[12,13] Whether the speaker considers another person talking to be overlapping or interrupting depends partly on culture. For example, many Italians, Asians, and Filipinos value talking together.[12,13]

🧩 NURSES AND INTERRUPTION

To communicate with patient safety in mind, you need to aim for a balanced conversation. If the patient overlaps you in conversation, then you can overlap, too. If the patient does not overlap, let the patient speak alone. You will need to develop the sensitivity to discern a patient's preferences for overlapping or speaking alone.

If you feel you are being interrupted, you must learn to speak up and say, in a calm and quiet voice "I'm getting to that, please let me finish what I was saying."

Listener Versus Information Provider

Many women typically listen more, whereas many men typically seek opportunities to give information. With one person talking and the other person listening, an unbalanced relationship occurs, with the giver of information having a higher status than the listener.[12,13] When men speak to each other, they may try to challenge the content of the message, match information given with their own expertise in the area, or sidetrack the speaker to a different topic. Men may view these behaviors as an exchange of information between two equals. In contrast, women may view challenges and sidetracks as rude, nonlistening behaviors that will break down relationships. Thus, women and men may be mutually dissatisfied with the arrangement of women typically listening and men typically providing information.[12,13]

Many women are more inclined to give listening responses, murmuring "yes" as encouragement for the speaker to continue and nodding the head to provide feedback and encourage a relationship. In contrast, men typically focus on the message and its literal meanings and will say what they mean in return. Therefore, men say "yes" and nod only if they agree.[12,13] Women also tend to ask more questions than men to encourage further verbal expressions. Women may attempt to draw quieter members of a group into a conversation, whereas men may assume that anyone who has something to say will volunteer it.[20]

 ## NURSES AND LISTENING VERSUS PROVIDING INFORMATION

To have patient-safe communication, you must learn to listen actively and also to provide information. Listening is a crucial skill. Listening responses—such as nodding your head or saying "yes" or "go on" as a patient speaks—are an effective means of showing a patient that you are interested and that you want the patient to continue talking.

In contrast, if you find yourself talking and the patient is doing all of the listening, the conversation is out of balance. Stop talking, and ask the patient for his ideas or opinions to draw him into the conversation

Storytelling

Most people, regardless of gender, like to tell stories. Storytelling involves exchanging accounts of personal experiences. The stories that women tell tend to revolve around relationships. Women prefer to tell stories of peculiar people and dramatize abnormal behavior.[12,13] Men typically like to tell stories of human contests.[12,13] They tell stories of how they acted alone and report a happy outcome in an adventure in which they came out on top.

By listening to patients' stories, you can help distract them from their problems. Other patient-safe communication interventions involving storytelling include reminiscence and life review, in which the patient recalls and talks about past life experiences. Through reminiscence and life reviews, patients learn to deal with crises and losses, prevent and reduce depression, and increase life satisfaction.[21,22]

GENDER DIFFERENCES IN LANGUAGE USE

In addition to the gender differences discussed so far, men and women may show varying patterns when it comes to specific language usage, such as using tag questions and conversational rituals.[12,13]

Tag Questions

Women tend to ask more questions than men, commonly in the form of tag questions.[12,13] The speaker adds a phrase at the end of a statement that turns it into a question: "I'd like to go out to eat—wouldn't you?" Women may use this form to hear the other's thoughts on the subject and encourage the expression of opinions. If the woman specifically wants to go out to dinner, however, she should make a statement such as, "I'd like to go out to dinner tonight."

The danger of tag questions is that the other person, especially a man, not aware of the purpose of the tag question, may answer with a personal opinion such as "I'd rather stay in tonight." If he had known that the speaker really wanted to go out, he might have gone along happily. Men are sometimes prone to respond more literally to questions and, therefore, may misinterpret some forms of questions.[12,13]

Another phrase used as a tag is, "What do you think?" The purpose is to make others feel involved and obtain opinions before making a decision. A problem occurs, however, if the person to whom the tag question is directed interprets this to mean, "Make the decision for me." The tag question may give the impression that the speaker lacks the confidence to make the decision.

Many women also ask "why" questions more often than men. They seek an explanation, perhaps in an attempt to understand the other's thoughts on the subject. The net effect of tag questions during conversations is that women may appear less intelligent or more uncertain.[12,13]

Nursing and Tag Questions

Your ability to ask questions is very important in allowing you to develop a better understanding of a situation and to devise solutions to problems. Tag questions typically are not useful, however. Instead of a tag question, make a direct and polite statement about what you would like to be done. For example, in a nursing home, a statement and tag question can get you into trouble. "It's time for your bath, don't you think?" may result in the patient saying, "No, I think I want to skip it today." If you really want something to get done right away because of the schedule, do not ask a question, make a statement. Do not give a person a choice if there really is none.

Conversational Rituals

Many women aim to be liked by peers, so in addition to tag questions they use conversational rituals. The rituals of women focus on establishing symmetrical connections in relationships because of a need to be closely affiliated with peers. Many women attempt to maintain equality, make other people feel comfortable, look closely at the effects of conversations on a person's verbal and nonverbal behaviors, and maintain attention to details.[12,13]

For example, many women say "I'm sorry" as a way of showing empathy and restoring balance to a conversation, not intending it to mean that they did something wrong. To some men, the woman who uses this phrase often may appear powerless.[12,13] Another ritual for many women is use of the word "thanks," tacked on to the end of a conversation, although there may be nothing specific to be thankful about. It is seen as a way of showing concern for others' feelings or work and also as thanking others for their time. A man may wonder, "Why is she thanking me?" [12,13]

A third ritual used by women is giving praise through compliments.[12,13] Women offer more compliments than men, and they give far more compliments to other women than they do to men. By so doing, they are attempting to promote group harmony.

Men also use conversational rituals, many of which relate to status. Male rituals involve joking, sarcasm, teasing, and playful put-downs.[12,13] To men, joking and teasing are part of the contest for status and a way of getting attention from others. Joking and teasing may also help avoid confronting an issue in an open manner. Women typically tell fewer jokes than men and often do not find teasing, sarcasm, and put-downs funny.[12,13]

NURSES AND RITUALS

Examine your use of rituals. If you hear yourself saying, "I'm sorry," "Thank you," or offering compliments frequently and without good reason, stop doing so. In addition, examine your use of joking. It can be useful in establishing rapport because everyone likes to laugh, but sarcasm, teasing, and put-downs may not be taken as humorous. The use of humor within nurse-patient relationships is the focus of Chapter 9.

Gender Differences in Nonverbal Behavior

Both male and female body language can be misinterpreted. Many women tend to have less confident body language and posture than men. Many women have been noted to take up less space, invade personal space less often, gesture more fluidly, and lower their eyes more in a negative encounter. This gives the impression of insecurity. They may also open their eyes wide to make a point, giving the impression of being naïve.[20,23] Women also smile and nod their heads more than men do. They tend to sit closer and look directly at each other as they speak.[12,13]

Many men, on the other hand, typically do not make direct facial contact with their eyes. They sit farther apart, at angles, and do not look at each other. To women, this gives the impression that men are not paying attention or do not think the conversation is important. Men also touch women more often than women touch men.[23,24]

Nurses and Body Language

Patients watch your body language closely, whether they know it or not. You must learn to project confidence and interest through your body language. Sit or stand 2 to 4 feet from the person, face the person directly as you speak, and look into the patient's eyes as you ask, "How are you doing today?" Listen carefully. Watch the nonverbal behaviors. Smile and nod your head, as appropriate, in response to what the patient tells you. Touch is a special form of patient-safe communication involving body language and is the subject of Chapter 8.

Gender Responses to Discomfort

Of special concern to nurses are gender differences in responding to discomfort and physical health problems.[25,26] Women are typically more expressive of discomforts and ask more questions than men. Men may not volunteer information; during interviews, you may need to question them carefully to obtain the details of a problem. All patients, regardless of setting, should be carefully instructed to report discomforts and encouraged to take pain medications.

CHAPTER SUMMARY

As a nurse, you need to become aware of communication differences based on gender and cultural contexts so that you can clearly deliver and decipher messages leading to positive transformational outcomes. First, you must become aware of how your own cultural and gender values, attitudes, and practices affect communication safety in patient and interdisciplinary relationships. Then, the patient's cultural and gender beliefs must be assessed and taken into consideration to form trusting interpersonal relationships, plan and implement care, and prevent patient harm. There will be differences in the selection of treatment modalities and the management of treatment plans based on your accurate assessment and understanding of the impact of cultural and gender values, attitudes, and practices of each patient. Health-care providers need to learn to conduct a cultural and gender context assessment and then analyze and solve health-care problems of patients and their family members from the patient's cultural and gender contextual perspective.

BUILDING HIGH-LEVEL COMMUNICATION COMPETENCE

For additional exercises, visit DavisPlus at http://davisplus.fadavis.com

1. **Cultural Self-Assessment.** Complete the brief cultural assessment below to help yourself become aware of your own cultural values, attitudes, and practices and how these affect your communication with patients and families. After you answer the questions, ask the questions of your parents and, if possible, your grandparents. Compare and contrast your answers with those of your classmates.

• To what culture and ethnic groups do you belong?

• In what country were you born?

• In what country were your ancestors born? (From what country or continent does your family originate?)

• Do you follow any traditions passed down to your generation? Give examples. What holidays do you celebrate, and what do you eat?

• Whom do you consider family members?

• In your family, who takes care of infants and children?

• In your family, who stays home from work and takes care of family members when they are sick?

• How are decisions made in your family?

• Where are your most elderly family members living?

• What happens to family members when they die?

• Who does what tasks in your family, such as preparing meals, cleaning the house, doing yard work?

• How important is it to be punctual?

• Is the gender of a baby important? Are girl and boy infants treated differently?

• What rules govern sexual activity for a man? a woman?

2. **Critical Thinking.** Give examples of communication strategies to use when a male nurse is assigned to give care to an 85-year-old female patient with severe arthritis, or when a female nurse is assigned to give care to an 85-year-old male patient with severe arthritis. How would you engage the patient?

References

1. McFarland, M., Wehbe-Alamah, H., Andrews, M., et al. Indigenous Transcultural Nursing Knowledge Discovered in a Metasynthesis of Culture Care Research Findings. Proceedings From 34th Annual Conference of the Transcultural Nursing Society, Sept. 24-27, 2008, Minneapolis, Minn.
2. Murphy, S.C. Mapping the Literature of Transcultural Nursing. Journal of the Medical Library Association. 94: E143-E151, 2006. Located at http://www.pubmedcentral.nih.gov/articlerender.fcgi?artid=1463039 Accessed October 2008.
3a. Kohls, R.L. Why Do Americans Act Like That? A Guide to Understand the U.S. Culture and its Values. Dr. L. Robert Kohls, Director of International Programs at San Francisco State University. Located at http://www.uku.fi/~paganuzz/xcult/values/Amer_values.htm Accessed October, 2008.
3b. Kohls, L.R. The Values Americans Live By. Located at http://web1.msue.msu.edu/intext/global/americanvalues.pdf Accessed October, 2008.
4. Purnell, L.D., Paulanka, B.J. Transcultural Health Care: A Culturally Competent Approach, 3rd ed. Philadelphia, F.A. Davis: 2008.
5. Purnell, L.D. Guide to Culturally Competent Health Care, 2nd ed. Philadelphia, F.A. Davis: 2009.
6. World Health Organization. Gender, Women, and Health. Located at http://www.who.int/gender/en/ Accessed October, 2008.
7. Brannon, L: Gender: Psychological Perspectives, 5th ed. Boston, Allyn & Bacon: 2007.
8. Moir, A., Jessel, D. Brain Sex: The Real Difference Between Men and Women. Seacaucus, N.J., Carole Publishing Group: 1991.
9. Gorski, R.A. Sexual Differentiation of the Endocrine Brain and Its Control Brain Endocrinology, ed 2. N.Y.,Raven Press: 1991.
10. Lehne, R.A. Pharmacology for Nursing Care, ed 4. Philadelphia, W.B. Saunders: 2006.
11. Gerlach, P.K. Gender and Communication: Typical Female/Male Differences in Priorities. Located at http://sfhelp.org/02/gender.htm Accessed October, 2008 .
12. Tannen, D. You Just Don't Understand: Women and Men in Conversation. N.Y.,Quill, Harper/Collins: 2001.
13. Tannen, D. Can't We Talk? Condensed from You Just Don't Understand. Located at http://raysweb.net/poems/articles/tannen.html Accessed October, 2008.
14. Hyde, J.S. Half the Human Experience: The Psychology of Women, 7th ed. Boston, Houghton-Mifflin: 2007.
15. Hyde, J.S. New Directions in the Study of Gender Similarities and Differences. Current Directions in Psychological Science 1:259-263, 2007.
16. Hyde, J.S., DeLamater, J.D.: Understanding Human Sexuality, 10th ed. N.Y., McGraw-Hill: 2008.
17. Else-Quest, N.M., Hyde, J.S., Goldsmith, H.H., et al. Gender Differences in Temperament: A Meta-Analysis. Psychological Bulletin 132:33-72, 2006.
18. Trossman, S. The Human Connection: Nurses and Their Patients. The American Nurse 30:1, 1998.
19. Lever, J. Sex Differences in the Complexity of Children's Play and Games. American Sociological Review 43:471, 1978.
20. Glass, L. He Says, She Says: Closing the Communication Gap Between the Sexes. N.Y., Perigree Books, Putnam Publishing Group: 1993.
21. Burnside, I., Haight, B. Reminiscence and Life Review: Therapeutic Interventions for Older People. Nurse Practitioner 19:55, 1994.
22. Schweitzer, P., Bruce, E. Remembering Yesterday, Caring Today: Reminiscence in Dementia Care: A Guide to Good Practice. London, Jessica Kingsley Publishers: 2008.
23. Glass, L. I Know What You're Thinking: Using the Four Codes of Reading People to Improve Your Life. Hoboken, N.J., John Wiley & Sons: 2003.
24. Aries, E: Gender and Communication. In Shaver, P., Hendrick, C. (eds.): Sex and Gender. Newbury Park, Calif., Sage: 1987, pp 149-176.
25. Verbrugge, L.M. Gender and Health: An Update on Hypotheses and Evidence. Journal of Health and Social Behavior 26:156, 1985.
26. Verbrugge, L.M. The Twain Meet: Empirical Explanations of Sex Differences in Health and Mortality. Journal of Health and Social Behavior 30:282, 1989.

2

Nurse-Patient Communication: Patient-Safe Communication in Professional Relationships

CHAPTER

6

Introduction to Nurse-Patient Relationships

Learning Outcomes

Upon completion of this chapter, you will be able to:

1. Identity the phases of the nurse-patient relationship.
2. Describe the relationship of the Transformational Model of Communication to the Patient-Safe Communication Process.
3. Examine the patient-safe communication process as a patient-safe strategy to prevent patient harm.
4. Explain the importance of developing collaborative relations with patients, their families, and legal guardians to establish mutual goals and objectives in nurse-patient relationships.
5. Describe the four universal communication styles that patients may use to respond to stressful situations.
6. Describe the importance of patient-safe strategies of assertiveness and professional identity management to manage stress in nurse-patient relationships.

Key Terms

Preorientation phase
Orientation phase
Working phase
Termination phase
Patient-safe communication process
Professional identity management

Stress
Blamer
Placator
Computer
Distractor
Assertivenss

The developing nurse communicator must now transition from understanding the basics of communication and interpersonal relationships into the high-level communication competency needed to develop and maintain the nurse-patient relationship. *For an interactive version of this activity, see DavisPlus at http://davisplus.fadavis.com.* You can complete an assessment of your current style of communication in relationships. This chapter describes the high-level communication competency needed in nurse-patient relationships.

In nurse-patient relationships, nurses attempt to develop collaborative relationships with patients, patient families, and legal guardians to establish mutual health-care goals and objectives. The nurse-patient relationship always includes the patient and will also include the legal guardians if the patient is younger than 18 or is otherwise unable to make decisions due to the nature of the health state. There are four phases of the nurse-patient relationship, as detailed in Box 6.1.

BOX 6.1 *Phases of the Nurse-Patient Relationship*

The nurse-patient relationship is a helping relationship.[1] The nurse must understand the phases of helping relationships in order to communicate effectively with patients and family members or guardians. Peplau described the phases as preinteraction, orientation, working, and termination.

Preinteraction occurs prior to meeting a patient; the nurse reviews available data on the patient to anticipate health needs and formulate a preliminary plan of care.

During *orientation,* the nurse and patient meet and get to know each other. This phase begins as an interpersonal relationship that lays the foundation for a nurse-patient relationship. Social greetings are followed by focusing on the reason for the need for patient care. The patient must be informed about what to expect and when the relationship will be terminated. The patient's problems and goals must be prioritized in collaboration with the nurse.

Next is the *working* phase, where the patient and nurse work together to attain mutual goals.

Last is the *termination* phase, focused on a smooth transition as care is passed to other caregivers. The nurse and patient evaluate goal achievement during the time they have worked together. The nurse reminds the patient ahead of time that he or she is leaving soon and then says goodbye.

High-level communication competency behaviors include communication knowledge, skill, and motivation.[2] Communication knowledge means knowing what behavior is best suited for a given situation. Communication skill is having the ability to apply the behavior in the given context. Communication motivation is having the desire to communicate in a highly competent manner.

HIGH-LEVEL COMMUNICATION COMPETENCY USING THE PATIENT-SAFE COMMUNICATION PROCESS

To help you achieve professional high-level communication competency in nurse-patient relationships, we have developed a systematic, decision-making Patient-Safe Communication Process. It is the key patient-safe communication strategy for appropriate and effective communication. The Patient-Safe Communication Process is derived from the transformational model, which is a *model of communicating competently,* with practical application to nurse-patient relationships as shown in Figure 6.1.

The Patient-Safe Communication Process takes into account the many variables that are risk factors for effective communication and the coordination of complex, interdependent, and dynamic activities required for effective communication to take place. In nurse-patient relationships, nurses and patients simultaneously send and receive messages and perform numerous perceptual, cognitive, and behavioral activities requiring communication to prevent harm to patients.

Communication Safety Alert

Nurses must strive to produce accurate messages through deliberate choices, monitor the emotions and reactions of patients, interpret the rapid stream of information, adjust choices to meet the situation, respond to changes in context, and preserve intended health goals and objectives as they collaborate with patients in an attempt to attain positive transformations.[3]

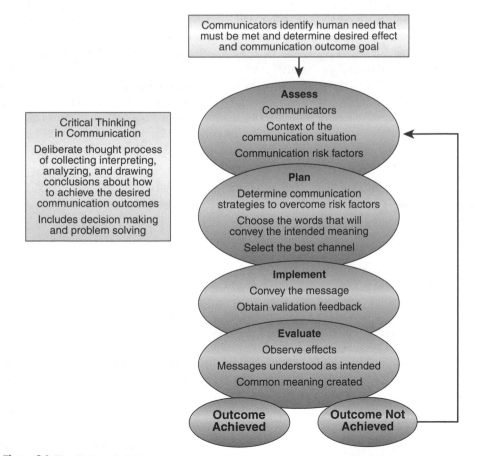

Figure 6.1 The Patient-Safe Communication Process.

Attaining Positive Transformations in Patients

Patient-safe communication within the nurse-patient relationship is transformational because the nurse and patient continue to grow and evolve based on the nature of communications about the health state of the patient. Communication changes both the nurse and patient from the person they were prior to the communication experience. Both the nurse and patient have effects on each other and transform each other through communication. If the nurse-patient relationship is successful, then the desired health outcomes that are optimal for the context of the situation will be achieved. If outcomes are not achieved, then the situation requires further assessment, planning, implementation, and evaluation, as depicted by the large circular arrow on the right of the diagram of the patient-safe process.

Nurse-patient communications differ from the communications that take place between you and other patient care providers, and it differs from your day-to-day interpersonal communications outside the patient care system. The difference is that patients have unmet safety and security needs because of alterations in health state. Patients are in a vulnerable position because they are no longer capable of independent self-care, and they are often dependent on patient care providers whom they do not know personally. Patients seek the assistance of patient care providers to prevent health problems, to detect and treat acute and chronic health problems, and when no more can be done, to find a way to die peacefully. Health concerns are very personal and private matters to resolve. Managing health concerns can become frustrating and upsetting to patients and families and can affect the way in which they communicate.

The patient-safe communication process enables you to engage the patient to the highest degree possible—given the patient's ability—and collaboratively work with the patient toward the attainment of health goals and objectives. The patient's health outcomes depend largely on your ability to communicate with the patient and other members of the health-care team. Health-care team communications are described in Chapters 12 and 13.

Communication Safety Alert

The patient-safe communication process leads to the recognition of needs, the establishment of mutual goals, and formation of trusting and collaborative nurse-patient relationships.

The nurse-patient relationship flowchart in Figure 6.2 contrasts nurse-patient communications that result in collaboration compared to those that result in conflict between the nurse and patient. If communication is not effective, conflict develops over health goals and objectives, and the amount of shared information will decrease, thereby increasing the likelihood of harmful events.

As shown in the flowchart, the nurse goes into a patient care situation with a preconceived set of goals and objectives that the nurse believes need to be achieved for an optimal health outcome. Likewise, the patient has a set of goals and objectives that she believes must be achieved for an optimal health outcome. These goals and objectives may not be the same.

During your first and subsequent encounters with a patient, you will communicate to establish mutual goals and objectives regarding patient care needs. Differing ideas about

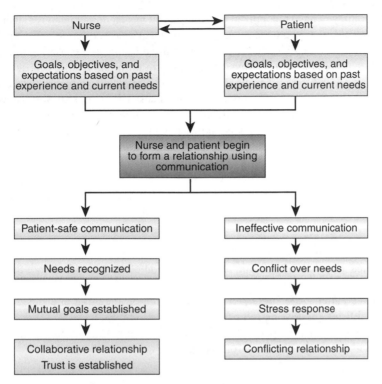

Figure 6.2 Flowchart of nurse-patient relationship.

the goals and objectives and disagreement regarding needs leads to conflict between the nurse and patient. Consequently, you and the patient will feel stress.

For example, suppose your goal is to prevent the complications of immobility for an elderly patient in a nursing home. You go into his room to get him out of bed for breakfast. The patient acts very sleepy and says, "I do not want to get up. Let me sleep." You know that trays are coming in 20 minutes and that the patient is scheduled to be in physical therapy in an hour.

You feel stress because you and the patient are not in agreement, and you need to establish a collaborative relationship with the patient. Use the patient-safe communication process as follows:

1. Assess the communicator to identify human needs: this person wants sleep, which is a very basic physical need.
2. Identify conflicting goals: patient wants to sleep; you want him up for physical therapy.
3. Respond with the patient-safe strategy of empathy to verify and clarify your assigned meaning to the situation: Empathically say, "You are tired today. How did you sleep last night?" He responds with, "The patient across the hall was making noise all night."
4. Respond with the patient-safe strategy of humor and use a joking tone of voice to say: "I guess the staff should have passed out ear plugs last night."
5. Evaluate creation of common meaning: the patient smiles a little and says, "You can say that again!"

At this point, you have recognized that the patient has an unmet need for sleep, and you have communicated that you understand his need and attained common meaning. Now you can negotiate a plan for activity and rest, saying: "Breakfast trays are coming in 20 minutes, and you have an appointment in Physical Therapy in an hour. Would you like 5 minutes more to sleep now, and then I'll come to get you up? There's also a period between therapy and lunch when you can take a nap when you get back. I'll hang a do-not-disturb sign on your door if you'd like." You must create common meaning that the need for sleep will be met. If you can negotiate mutual understanding and create common meaning in developing a workable plan of action with the patient's cooperation, there is increased liklihood of attaining positive health outcomes and positive transformations.

Once you negotiate an action plan with the patient, however, you must follow through. You told him he could have a nap, so make sure he gets one. That way, the patient will learn to trust you because you are reliable. This example of the patient-safe communication process:

- Recognizes differences in patient and nurse expectations
- Demonstrates the use of verifcation and clarification of messages between the nurse and patient
- Demonstrates patient-safe strategies to create common meaning and put the patient at ease by establishing a trusting relationship
- Illustrates how to enlist the patient's cooperation in negotiating mutual goals and objectives that will lead to postive transformations

Communication Safety Alert

No matter what the activities the nurse hopes to accomplish with the patient, use the patient-safe communication process for the highest probablity of attaining common meaning and positive health transformations.

Understanding the Patient's Viewpoint and the Situational Context

The nurse must strive to understand a situation from the patient's viewpoint. How does the patient perceive the situation, and how is it similar to or different from the perceptions you hold as the patient care provider? What is the impact of the patient's self-esteem and self-concept? What are the effects of gender differences in communication or culturally derived feelings, beliefs, attitudes, and values? Nurses assess the impact of life experiences; social, cultural, and environmental backgrounds; gender issues; self-esteem; and self-concept, all of which affect the interaction with the patient.

In general, the better the match between the backgrounds of the patient and the nurse, the easier it is to communicate. For example, as a student nurse your clinical group is providing care to patients and families in a hospice house. The patients and families are from different religious backgrounds. You would probably feel most comfortable if your assignment was a patient whose background is similar to your own because it would be easiest to understand the customs, practices, and beliefs of the dying patient and the surrounding family members. It would be much more difficult to anticipate the spiritual needs of a patient and family from a culture unfamiliar to you.

Communication Safety Alert

Two patients scheduled for the same test or procedure are likely to respond differently to the health-care situation, based on previous life experiences and biological, psychological, social, and cultural differences that were described in Unit 1.

✦ COMMUNICATING WITH PATIENTS WITH COGNITIVE, VISUAL, OR AUDITORY IMPAIRMENTS

Understanding the patients' viewpoint and the situational context can become very challenging and stressful when the patient has cognitive impairments, such as Alzeimer's disease or other forms of dementia and brain damage. The patient has difficulty understanding what is said, expressing thoughts and feelings, and may be feeling lonely, isolated, and fearful. The patient may have difficulty finding the right words, may easily lose a train of thought, or have difficulty organizing words logically. The patient may use familiar words repeatedly or invent new words to describe familiar things. Alternately, the patient may speak less often or rely on gestures intead of speaking. As dementia progresses, communication can become more challenging. There are patient-safe communication strategies to communicate with patients who have cognitive, hearing, or vision impairments. See *DavisPlus* at *http://davisplus.fadavis.com* for the recommendations from the Alzheimer's Association[4] for communicating with patients with cognitive impairments, memory loss, and auditory or visual impairments.

✦ STRESS IN THE NURSE-PATIENT RELATIONSHIP

Nurses strive to understand the health-care situation from the patient's perspective and from within situational contexts. Additionally, nurses realize that health-care situations are stressful for patients and families and that stress will have an impact on communication processes. In this next section, we describe universal communication styles patients may use when they are feeling stressed, and then we introduce two patient-safe nursing strategies that include assertiveness and professional identity management that facilitate the maintainance of professional relationships.

When either person in a communication interaction is under stress, communication becomes more difficult. In patient care environments, there are many reasons for everyone to feel stressed—patients, families, and even the patient care providers themselves. The patients and families need to change their lives, at least temporarily, sometimes permanently, to adapt to health problems and related needs. Patient care providers are typically rushed because they are short-staffed. Patient care providers need to move on quickly to the next patient or to the seemingly unending pile of paperwork.

Communication Safety Alert

Virtually all patients and family members feel some degree of anxiety, tension, or fear as they face the stress of managing a patient care situation and interacting with patient care providers. The emotions of anxiety, tension, and fear are key communication risk factors that are present in many patient care situations. These emotions create stress in the nurse-patient relationship.

Stress, whether physical or emotional, causes the body to respond with a fight-or-flight reaction to the stressor. The theory of stress and seminal research on the fight-or-flight reaction have been credited to the psychologist Hans Selye.[5] During the fight-or-flight reaction, hormones are released that increase blood pressure, pulse, and breathing. The pupils dilate, and the palms sweat. A person's perception of environmental events creates stress, which leads to physiological reactions, with emotional and behavioral consequences.

This response occurs whenever a person's basic needs are not met. Basic needs that could be threatened during stressful situations have been categorized by Maslow, who developed the classic basic human needs theory.[6] He categorized basic human needs as safety and security, love and belonging, self-esteem, and physiological. Some or all of these categories of needs may be threatened as a result of a health problem.

In response to stress, people react emotionally and behaviorally. The feelings that accompany the situation are very uncomfortable. The person feels anxious, nervous, and tense; may be irritable; may not sleep well, get headaches, or become nauseated. It is human nature to do something to relieve these feelings of stress and anxiety. For example, the person could talk, laugh, or cry.

Communication Safety Alert

It is also important for you to understand your own typical response style when you are under stress. Patient care situations can be very stressful for you, the nurse, as well as for patients and their families.

Understanding Physical and Emotional Responses to Stress

Nurses must understand the diagnosis and treatment of the patient's physical responses in patient care settings. For example, when a patient is in labor, you must know how to attach and interpret the fetal monitor. If the baby shows signs of distress, you will need to position the mother, start oxygen, start an intravenous line, and prepare for emergency delivery, if necessary. Obviously, when it comes to physical care for a patient, knowing what to do and how to do it are essential to your success as a nurse.

Just as important, however, is your ability to analyze, understand, and intervene in response to the emotional conditions of patients and their families in patient care situations. Analyzing and intervening with emotional responses is another primary goal of nursing care, and it requires high-level communication competency. For example, every mother wonders if she and her child are going to make it through the delivery. Even the most rational pregnant woman, a woman who remembers that thousands of babies are born daily and that the odds favor everything coming out fine, may have some doubts that cause her tension and anxiety.

Near the end of labor, the woman has painful contractions that may cause her to lose control and cry. She may become short-tempered and snap at her partner or you because of her pain and anxiety. To communicate with this anxious, laboring woman, speak slowly, clearly, and calmly as you provide pain control measures and help the woman breathe properly.

In this situation, you would communicate with this woman by coaching her through each contraction, giving specific directions and demonstrating what should be done as needed. At the same time, you would offer reassurance that everything is progressing normally, that fetal heart rate patterns show the baby is doing well, and the baby will be born soon.

Nurses strive to promote optimal physical and emotional positive transformational outcomes. As a nurse, you must know what to say to patients as you administer physical care so that you can also ease the emotional stress the patient feels. Patient care settings are often both physically and emotionally threatening. By easing the patient's emotional stress, you enable the patient to cope effectively with the situation and can improve the emotional comfort level.[7] When you find yourself in a difficult communication situation in which emotions are tense, the patient-safe communication process can help facilitate optimal transformational outcomes.

Communication Safety Alert

Patients feel threatened when they believe they are not understood or when they do not understand what is happening to them, and they react physically and emotionally to the situation. If you fail to communicate effectively to establish a collaborative relationship early in such a situation, patients and families can become very distressed. Any time a patient is acting distressed, you should assume that needs are not being met and use the patient-safe communication process to establish a collaborative relationship.

Universal Responses to Stress

Virginia Satir has researched and developed a classic theory of four universal communication styles that many people use to respond to stressful situations when their self-esteem is threatened.[8,9] You must learn to recognize each of these communication styles in the nurse-patient relationship: blamer, placater, computer, and distracter.

Blamer. Imagine you are going into the room of a blamer to complete the morning assessment. You wake the patient gently, but much to your surprise, the patient starts pointing his finger and says loudly, "Nobody cares what I want!" or "You always come to check my blood pressure when I'm sleeping. Can't you see I'm sleeping? What's wrong with you?" All you did was to wake him to do the morning assessment that had to be done because he had surgery less than 24 hours ago. You never even met him. The blamer uses accusatory "you" statements, sarcasm, put-downs, expressions of superiority, and loaded words intended to start fights. The blamer may interrupt, yell, call names, demand, give orders, ignore people, hang up on phone conversations, and walk away when someone is talking.

Placater. You go into the next room to ask the patient if she has decided on the rehabilitation center where she would like to be transferred because she needs extensive physical therapy. She had a bad fall and broke her hip. Her family cannot take care of her at home until she can do more for herself. When you ask the question, the patient fidgets and picks at her fingernails. With a pleading look in her eyes and a soft voice, she says "I do not care . . . er, what do you think? My son wants me to go to Parkside, but my daughter says I should go to Hillsville near her home. I'm sorry, but I do not know what to do." The placater has a hard time making decisions, may make numerous apologies, and stumble in coming to the point. The placater is frightened of offending or angering anyone, goes along with others when she or he really does not want to, apologizes for things he or she did not do, decides that he or she cannot do something before trying it, and says yes when he or she really means no.

Computer. Out in the hall, you run into the patient's son, who when under stress responds in the computer style. You say, "Your mother is upset about where she should go for rehabilitation. She seems to be torn between the place you believe is best and the place your sister feels is best." He replies with a monotone, matter-of-fact voice, "There's a simple solution to the problem. No rational person would need to get upset about it." The computer does not want to reveal feelings and resists discussing them when asked, usually out of fear that doing so is a sign of weakness. This person is quiet, aloof, reserved, and withdrawn and has difficulty responding when others express their feelings.

Distracter. Just then, the patient's daughter, a distracter, approaches you in the hallway. You explain that her mother is upset about where she should go for rehabilitation. She turns to her brother, points a finger at him, and says, "You always want things your way!" Then she turns to you with quiet, downcast eyes and says, "Whatever Mother wants, I really do not care. There should be an easy answer to the problem." A distracter jumps from one style (blamer, placater, or computer) to another, following random urges about what to say. The distracter talks nervously, making little sense, expending energy but failing to focus on the problem or how to solve it.

Some patients are bound in these styles of behavior because they have used them for years to deal with stress and anxiety. When interacting with patients and their families in stressful situations, it is up to you to remain in control to be able to respond effectively and carry out your role.

How you present yourself to others as you respond to stressful situations is extremely important. Two very important patient-safe strategies you must use are: assertiveness and management of professional identity.

Assertiveness

As a professional nurse, you must learn to become assertive. The assertive nurse is confident and speaks up, asks for information or cooperation clearly, and can say no to requests without feeling guilty. The assertive nurse makes honest statements that are direct; keeps a relaxed and open posture; maintains direct eye contact, and hand gestures and body movements are slow and relaxed. An assertive nurse can control her or his temper when people get angry and start to yell and asks questions to understand and analyze a situation.[10] Using assertiveness as a patient-safe strategy takes practice.

We all need to please others, criticize others, defend ourselves, and use our intellect to explain to others and change the subject when appropriate. An assertive person can accomplish all these things. You apologize for something you have done incorrectly or failed to do. When you criticize, you evaluate an act rather than blame the person, and you make suggestions for better future performances. You can show your feelings as you give an explanation. You can also clearly say that you need to change the subject witout confusing the other person as to what you are talking about.

To manage the stressful situation described earlier, use a clear, firm, relaxed voice as you summarize the situation as you see it. You could say, "Your mother needs to make a decision about where to go for rehabilitation. Let's go discuss with your mother the advantages and disadvantages of each of the places that are suited to meet her needs. She needs support from both of you on whatever she decides." In so doing, this nurse has been assertive, direct, and to the point. In addition, nurses use their appearance, mannerisms, and control of the setting to manage stressful situations. This is known as management of professional identity in the nurse-patient relationship.

Management of Professional Identity

Patients respond to the nurse's professional identity, so it is very important to understand that identity management is a communication strategy used by high-level communicators to present themselves to others and influence how others form perceptions and impressions about them.[11] The presenting self is the way you present yourself to others and the impressions others form as a result.[12] It is the presenting self that individuals attempt to manage carefully as highly competent communicators.

Goffman[13] described the identity we present to others using the term *face* to refer to our socially approved identity. Consider the face or the image of yourself you present at an interview or in a courtroom. You adjust your style of attire, tone of voice, gestures, and the words that you use. Think about the way you would present yourself as a nurse in the clinical setting. It is different from the way you would present yourself at a family celebration. "Putting on a face" is the classic expression that exemplifies the communication strategy of managing identity.

Individuals are motivated to manage their identities to achieve desired communication outcomes to meet human needs, professional goals, and the needs of others. Each of us has a repertoire of faces, depending on the desired outcome. We become skilled in selecting the face, or image, we choose to project as appropriate for the setting and context. We put on a face and manage our identity through three mechanisms: mannerisms, appearance, and setting.[14]

Manners

We manage identity through the use of manners. We are socialized early in our lives to shape the opinions others will form of us. We may not have had to apply the same rules in the privacy and comfort of our home, but we still know to adapt our behavior in public. In nursing, the stakes are higher when it comes to manners and presenting ourselves to patients. We carefully choose how we conduct ourselves during professional relationships.

Some people are more aware of the manners they present than others. Those with high self-monitoring have greater ability to pay attention to their own behavior and the reactions of others, adjusting their communications to create the necessary impressions, intended effects, and desired outcomes. These individuals can appear interested when they are really feeling bored or listless and can handle social and professional situations well, often putting others at ease. Think about your manners as you conduct a health history, physical assessment, procedures, or patient teaching. Suppose you discover your patient is an alcoholic and abuses drugs. As an individual, you have the right to your opinions about risky health behaviors such as alcoholism and drug abuse; however, as a nurse, you do not have the right to express these views, verbally or nonverbally, to patients. You must keep moral judgments outside of the nurse-patient relationship. Patients are sensitive to your mannerisms and will gauge their sense of trust in you accordingly. If trust is missing, patient information will not be shared, resulting in patient harm.

Appearance

We manage identity through the use of appearance. Appearance refers to the personal items individuals use to shape an image.[11] Appearance includes a particular hair style, choice of makeup, and clothing. The professional dress of a nurse transmits powerful messages to patients, their families, colleagues, and the public at large. Managing appearance in nursing conveys nonverbal purposeful messages of a positive image of professionalism.

Patients perceive that when a nurse projects a positive professional appearance, it "communicates that the nurse cares about herself or himself; therefore, the impression is that he or she will 'take good care of me.'"[15]

In recent years, body adornment, including tattoos and facial and body piercing, have become increasingly popular. Tattoos and body piercing affect professional image negatively and may ultimately affect patient safety because "patients may have negative attitudes towards nurses with body adornment. To many, it demeans health care's professional image."[16]

Research demonstrates that health-care administrators hold similar negative views about people with tattoos.[17] "Although nurse managers cannot prohibit employees from getting tattoos or body piercings, they can establish dress codes that limit the amount of adornment that employees may display. Courts will uphold dress codes based on valid and nondiscriminatory reasons such as safety concerns, professionalism and business interests."[16]

A positive first impression is necessary to establish the nurse-patient relationship. How comfortable will your 80-year-old patient be in telling you of his fear that his medications are incorrect if you enter the room with your tongue and eyebrow pierced? If the patient does not trust you because of his impressions of you, you have effectively blocked communications and silenced the patient. You are no longer able to be patient-safe, and essential patient information may become inaccessible, thereby increasing the patient's risk for a harmful event. Use professional appearance as a means to nurture the communication situation and offer the best chance for patients to relate to you with trust and willingness to express their human needs. You will need to follow the dress code of your educational institution and the patient care workplaces.

In addition, first impressions also transmit powerful messages to a nursing manager. For example, you would not wear jeans and a sweatshirt to an interview. This would not be appropriate for the context of the situation and would not cast the professional image of a nurse you want to portray. A well-dressed appearance tends to convey a higher level of knowledge and a sincere interest in advancement. A disheveled worker, on the other hand, gives the impression of being a disinterested, marginal performer.[18]

Setting

We also manage identity through our choice of setting, which refers to the physical realm we use to influence others. In interpersonal relationships, setting includes, for example, the way we decorate our apartment or home. In nursing, it refers to the privacy we create for the patient when we are conducting a health history, obtaining informed consent, or performing an invasive procedure. Our ability to manipulate the setting is needed to create a safe, confidential environment. For example, nurses knock before entering a room and pull privacy curtains around the patient prior to performing procedures.

CHAPTER SUMMARY

Derived from the Transformational Model of Communication, the Patient-Safe Communication Process is described as an instrument for patient safety used to create trusting and collaborative relationships with patients and families in successful nurse-patient relationships. Failure to establish trust and collaboration will result in stress and conflict in the nurse-patient relationship. High-level communication competency involves the use of the Patient-Safe Communication Process, which includes assessing the patient, the context, and the risk factors; identifying the communication needs, goals, and desired outcomes; planning the message; implementing patient-safe communications strategies, and evaluating communication outcomes.

BUILDING HIGH-LEVEL COMMUNICATION COMPETENCY

For an interactive version of this activity, see DavisPlus at http://davisplus. fadavis.com

1. Recall a difficult communication you had recently with a patient. Think about the setting, the circumstances surrounding the conflict, and the reactions (verbal and nonverbal) of those involved. Now make a two-column table. In the first column, record your verbal and nonverbal messages. What got you upset? With which communication style did you react? What did you want for yourself? What did you want from the other person?

2. Use the Patient-Safe Communication Process to analyze the difficult communication situation described in Exercise 1. What could you have done to respond using patient-safe strategies?

References

1. Peplau, H. Interpersonal Relations in Nursing: A Conceptual Frame of Reference for Psychodynamic Nursing. N.Y., Macmillan/McGraw-Hill: 1988.
2. Spitzberg, B.H., Cupach, W.R.: Interpersonal Communication Competence. Beverly Hills, Calif., Sage: 1984.
3. Poole, M.S., Walther, J.B. National Communication Association. Communication—Ubiquitous, Complex, and Consequential. Washington, D.C., 2001. Located at http://www.natcom.org/research/monograph.pdf
4. Alzheimer's Association. Communication: Best Ways to Interact With the Person With Dementia. Located at www.alz.org Accessed April 3, 2009.
5. Selye, H. The Stress of Life. N.Y., McGraw-Hill: 1976.
6. Maslow, A. Motivation and Personality. N.Y., Harper & Row: 1970.
7. Williams, A.M., Irurita, V.F. Emotional Comfort: The Patient's Perspective of a Therapeutic Context. International Journal of Nursing Studies 43:405, 2006.
8. Satir, V. Conjoint Family Therapy. Palo Alto, Calif., Science and Behavior Books: 1964.
9. Satir, V. The New Peoplemaking. Mountain View, Calif., Science and Behavior Books: 1988.
10. Clark, C.C.: Holistic Assertiveness Skills for Nurses: Empower Yourself and Others. N.Y., Springer: 2003.
11. Adler, R.B., Rosenfeld, L.B., Proctor, R.F., et al. Interplay: The Process of Interpersonal Communication. Don Mills, Ontario, Canada, Oxford University Press: 2006.
12. Redhill, D. Ten Tips for Managing Your Corporate Identity. Workforce 78: 2, 1999.
13. Goffman, E. The Presentation of Self in Everyday Life. Garden City, N.Y., Doubleday: 1959.
14. Vander Zanden, J.W. Social Psychology, 3rd ed., N.Y.: Random House: 1984, pp. 235-237.
15. LaSala, K.B., Nelson, J. What Contributes to Professionalism? MEDSURG Nursing 14, 2005.
16. Smith, M.H. Body Adornment: Know the Limits. Nursing Management 34:22-24, 2003.
17. Stuppy, D., Armstrong, M., Casals-Ariet, C. Attitudes of Health Care Providers and Students Towards Tattooed People. Journal of Advanced Nursing. 27:1165-1170, 1998.
18. Townsel, L.J. Working Women: Dressing for Success. Ebony, 51:60-65, 1996.

CHAPTER 7

Patient Safety Risk Factors Affecting Communication Climates

Learning Outcomes

Upon completion of this chapter, you will be able to:

1. Identify transformational model risk factors that impede creation of common meaning and affect communication climates.
2. Define communication climates and describe how communication climates develop.
3. Identify the impact of illness on self-esteem and self-worth of the patient, family, and nurse and its effects on the communication climate.
4. Describe the physical and psychosocial stages of illness, grief, and loss affecting the communication climate.
5. Describe patient-safe strategies to create positive communication climates and change negative communication climates into positive ones.
6. Identify strategies to manage personal emotions.

Key Words

Communication climate
Confirming messages
Disconfirming messages
Save face

"I" statements
Progressive relaxation
Visual imagery

Communication climate is defined as the tone, emotions, and attitudes of individuals in relationships.[1] The communication climate is directly affected by the risk factors of the transformational model because risk factors have a negative impact on climate: the more risk factors, the more potential for a negative climate. Communication risk factors can distort clear communication by interfering with the exactness of the message, which results in misinterpretations, which lead to negative tones, emotions, and attitudes within the nurse-patient relationship. The negative tones, emotions, and attitudes create obstacles to negotiating common meaning between the nurse and patient and increase the likelihood that communicators will not achieve intended communication outcomes.

Risk factors fall into two categories—emotional and physiological—and the factors from both categories interact with each other.

- **Emotional risk factors:** Fear of the unknown, anxiety, grief and loss, dependency, sadness, pain, resentment, anger, insecurity, disbelief, and denial.
- **Physiological risk factors:** Physical disabilities, sensory impairment, sedation, memory loss, and fatigue.

This chapter examines these emotional and physiological contents of the risk factor ring of the Transformational Model of Communication shown in Chapter 2 and the impact of these risk factors on the communication climate within the nurse-patient relationship. To conclude this chapter, we will introduce what can be done to transform negative communication climates.

THE COMMUNICATION CLIMATE

Whenever walking into a room where there are two or more people communicating, it is very important to assess the communication climate *before* interrupting or joining the conversation.

How Communication Climates Develop

Communication climate reflects, in part, the level of self-esteem of all individuals in the context of a particular situation and refers to the social tone of relationships.[2] The social tone of a relationship, and the communication climate that tone sets, is determined by the feelings of worth individuals hold and the extent to which they see themselves as valued by others in the relationships or social group. Communicators who perceive they are valuable and liked by others help create a positive tone in relationships and a positive communication climate, whereas those who perceive themselves as unimportant, devalued, and not liked by others help create a negative tone and a negative communication climate.[2]

The tone of the message itself also plays a role in setting the communication climate. Individuals tend to respond in ways similar to the tone conveyed in messages.[3] In communications that convey warmth and sincerity, the communication climate will likely be warm and sincere. In communication where there is hostility and aggression, the communication climate will likely be hostile and aggressive.

Messages that convey that a person is important, worthy, or makes a difference are termed *confirming messages.*[2] Messages that convey that a person is unworthy, insignificant, and easily discounted are termed *disconfirming messages.*[2] The nurse needs to use a specific patient-safe strategy of confirming messages to create positive communication climates

Responding With Confirming Messages Promotes a Positive Communication Climate

Confirming messages are conveyed through five types of statements, including recognition, acknowledgment, endorsement, compliment, and empathy[4]:

- **Recognition:** The basic way to send confirming messages is to *recognize* another person. You recognize the person as someone worthy and important to you. This is observed when you smile or wave to someone and greet the person in a friendly and pleasant manner; the greeting is very important in setting the tone of a relationship.
- **Acknowledgment:** Acknowledging the strengths, talents, aspirations, and feelings of others confirms their self-value. Examples of acknowledgement messages include: "You make a really good point here."
- **Endorsement:** Endorsement is a proclamation that you agree with the thoughts of another. Endorsement can also be as subtle as nodding when another speaks or maintaining eye contact and demonstrating "leaning in" behavior.
- **Compliment:** When we make a special point to tell others that we like something they have done or something about them personally, we confirm their sense of worth.
- **Empathy:** When we perceive the life experiences and feelings of someone and talk about our perceptions with that person, we are using empathy. "I'll bet there are other things you'd rather be doing than lying in this bed with a fractured hip."

Responding With Disconfirming Messages Promotes a Negative Communication Climate

We send and receive disconfirming messages every day with friends and family. Such intermittent disconfirming messages usually do not affect the communication climate.[2] When disconfirming messages become a pattern of communication, however, a negative communication climate may develop. In nursing, we need to select our responses to patients carefully to avoid sending disconfirming messages that may endanger the development of trust in the nurse-patient relationship.

There are six types of disconfirming responses, including[5]:

- **Unreceptive responses:** This response fails to acknowledge the communicative attempt of another. Being unreceptive to the messages of others by avoiding eye contact or offering the silent treatment conveys a diminished value of another if done with the intent of discounting an individual. The nurse looks at the form she is completing and asks history questions without looking at the patient. Always use active listening, make eye contact, and pay careful attention to verbal and nonverbal behaviors. Provide feedback to complete the communication process when interacting with patients.
- **Interruption responses:** When we begin speaking before another has finished, our behavior sends a message of disconfirmation. Always use active listening, and allow patients to tell their story in their own words without interruption.
- **Irrelevant responses:** This is a response that has nothing to do with the subject being discussed. It signals others that you are not listening and sends a message that they are not important. Always use active listening, and carefully respond directly to the patient's request.
- **Tangential responses:** In this situation, you at least partially acknowledge another person, but are only minimally attending to the message. "Can you help me change my

gown?" asks the patient. Your response, "I really need to give you your medications." Be very direct, and let the patient know you will be back or that you will send someone to help.

- **Impersonal responses:** These responses are intellectualized or over-generalized statements that convey ambiguity in the communication situation and can disconfirm the value of another. For example, the patient tells the nurse he is having difficulty coping with the behaviors of his teenage son. The nurse responds, "Yes, it is a huge issue in today's world, isn't it? Every day, there is something in the news about problems with bringing up teenagers." Respond with encouraging statements. Use paraphrasing and empathy to facilitate nurse-patient communications and promote positive climates.

- **Ambiguous responses:** An ambiguous response contains more than one meaning and leaves communications unclear. People receiving these responses feel uncertain as to how they should assign meaning and can feel less valued. For example, a patient asks if you can do his dressing change before his family comes to visit, and you reply, "I'll see. That might work." Respond to patients with clear messages, and do not put them in a position to feel uncertain about the intended meaning of your message.

In addition, Adler[2] describes the following disconfirming response:

- **"You Are Wrong, and I am Right":** For example, "Mrs. Jones, you are completely wrong here in thinking your mother can return home. You have not considered any of her needs. You need to check into nursing home placement." There are times when we disagree, but a blunt response is not appropriate. It is possible to turn a "you are wrong, and I am right" message into a constructive one through learning to be tactful and saving face. Stated positively, the message would begin with an acknowledgement of the other, not a judgment against or attack on the individual, and deliver a sound argument in support of an opposing view. "Mrs. Jones, I see where you are going with this, and I like the idea of planning now for your mother's discharge; however, there are many things to consider in ensuring she is safe at home. We should examine all the requirements and take a look at our options for when she leaves the hospital." The key to maintaining positive climates is to confirm the worth of others. This includes addressing issues of disagreement objectively and ensuring that messages do not attack the individual personally.

Before we can begin to learn how to transform a negative climate, we need to have a thorough understanding of the nature of illness and how it threatens self-esteem, which influences the communication climate within nurse-patient relationships.

✚ ILLNESS: A THREAT TO SELF-ESTEEM FOR PATIENT, FAMILY, AND NURSE

Illness affects the communication climate because it threatens self-esteem and threatens feelings of self-worth.[6] More specifically, illness alters the tone, emotions, and attitudes of the patient, family, and nurse, resulting in high risk for developing negative communication climates. Alterations in self-esteem and feelings of value occur during illness because of numerous threats inherent to illness, such as threats to livelihood, role performance, and even life itself.

The type of illness and the person's perception of its implications are two important factors that bear on the severity of impact on self-esteem and self-value. For example, consider the 36-year-old woman who works as an elementary school teacher, has a husband and two young children, and has undergone a mastectomy. Her self-esteem is affected—profoundly—by the change in her body image resulting from the mastectomy. Her sense of value will be affected by her perceptions of her changed ability to perform her roles of teacher, wife, and mother.

You go into the room, and she and her husband are crying, and you immediately recognize the negative communication climate. As a nurse, the self-esteem and value you place on yourself may be affected by the tone, emotions, and attitudes in a negative climate. Tone, emotions, and attitudes are contagious. In general, you will feel anxious whenever you believe you should be able to respond appropriately in a nursing situation to create a positive communication climate, but you find that you cannot.

The way to reduce anxiety and build self-esteem in yourself in the face of negative communication climates is to develop knowledge and competence in managing emotional responses in patients, their families, and yourself.

Impact of Illness on Communication Climate: Physical and Psychosocial Stages

The types and the ramifications of illness that affect a patient's self-esteem and value involve two stages: physical and psychosocial.[7] Although these stages occur simultaneously, they are described separately here to facilitate your understanding of patient and family reactions to illness and the effect on the communication climate.

Physical Stages

The physical stages of illness are its onset, course, and prognosis. An illness may have gradual onset, with symptoms getting progressively worse, as in diabetes, or it may have a sudden onset, as in a head injury that results from a car accident. Course refers to the length of time the person has to alter her lifestyle to manage the problem. Prognosis refers to the expected outcome, such as complete recovery, chronic illness, or death. The physical states are clear and easily recognized.

Psychosocial Stages

Much more complicated than the physical stages are the psychosocial, emotion-laden stages of illness. The emotional response arises from damage to self-esteem and feelings of worthlessnes that are related to loss. The patient and family suffer losses when they may never be the same again as a result of the illness. The patient may lose a body part or a physiological function, such as the ability to have children after a hysterectomy. Illness may cause the patient to lose external possessions as well, such as a job. The patient and family may lose their home, for example, if illness requires that the patient be placed in a nursing home or extended-care facility. In addition, permanent neurological changes or death can take the patient away from the family. For many of the changes brought about by illness, patients and families gradually adjust to the losses and damage to self-esteem with the help of nurses who help transform negative communication climates and help patients and families attain and maintain positive communication climates.

Psychologically and socially, the patient and family assimilate the physical changes by going through three phases: a transition to illness, acceptance of the illness, and convalescence as the patient recovers.[7]

Transition to illness: The transition to illness is the time between the appearance of an illness (the onset) and the patient's admission to himself that he is indeed ill. The self-image of a healthy and vital person is being disrupted by symptoms. Denial and rationalization characterize this period; both are defenses against the threat to self-esteem. Both defenses come into play to avoid the emotions associated with becoming ill.

Acceptance: Acceptance begins at the point when the person has decided something is definitely wrong and needs to do something about it.

Convalescence: Convalescence begins once the patient is stabilized and starts to recover. Physically, the patient is getting better. Sadness and anger are prevalent in this stage. The patient may become frustrated and upset, especially if the illness is extended or severe. The limitations on functioning are the primary problem.

If the patient is dying, the family and patient will grieve and mourn the loss. Grief and mourning also occur when recovery from illness is incomplete; the patient experiences significant loss as a result of the health alteration.

Grief associated with death and significant loss initially produces shock, disbelief, and denial. As the loss begins to sink in, many people feel anger because they have no control over the situation. As a result, they may direct that anger at you or other health-care personnel. Next, they may express guilt and fear that they are being punished. Depression and sadness occur when the patient and family recognize that their lives will never again be the same. Finally, the patient and family come to terms with the loss and begin making plans for the future.[8,9a]

The Patient's Personal and Unique Response

Not everyone goes through each physical and psychosocial stage. Also, while in a stage, not everyone progresses at the same rate, and not everyone responds in the same way. People's responses depend on their previous experience with illness and the health-care system as well as on their biological, psychological, social, gender, and cultural differences as described in Unit 1. In general, the more severe the illness, the more extensive the emotional, behavioral, and physical response. Two patients who have the same diagnosis may respond quite differently.

Dependency: The Sick Role: Resentment, Anger

Once a person has been diagnosed as "sick" with a specific set of symptoms, society excuses the person from role responsibilities. Traditional North American cultural sick role beliefs assume that the sick person and family will seek out and collaborate fully with health-care professionals, who are supposed to know more than the patient and family about the health problem and how to correct it. It is assumed that the sick person wants to get well and will do everything as instructed by health-care providers to get better as quickly as possible.[9b]

For some people, the worst part of being sick is that they have to depend on others to take care of them. They cannot tolerate the thought that they are no longer independent and productive and, at least temporarily, that they have to give up social, professional, and community roles that are important to their self-esteem.

On the other end of the dependency continuum is the person who refuses to perform self-care activities even after physically recovering to the point of being able to perform them. This patient does not seem to want to give up the sick role; in fact, the patient may enjoy the attention being received from health-care professionals, family, and friends.

This attitude reflects low self-esteem. In addition, some patients may also feel insecure and incapable of doing things on their own, even though they have recovered physically.

 TRANSFORMING NEGATIVE COMMUNICATION
CLIMATES TO POSITIVE ONES

Emotional Release

Nurses must do all they can to promote a postive communication climate and to transform negative climates into positive ones. A very important patient-safe communication strategy is to acknowledge and accept emotions through use of empathy and active listening responses.

Communication Safety Alert

Emotions are real and must be recognized and acknowledged by the nurse. If the patient seems upset to you, clarify and verify by making a verbal observation and asking what is wrong through use of the patient-safe strategy of perception checking: "You seem a little down today, is something bothering you?" Patient-safe communication in emotional situations is intended to facilitate the expression of the emotion and to talk with the patient about concerns.

Encourage patients to express their emotions. Patients or family members may talk angrily or cry when they are discouraged, frustrated, or upset. Alternatively, they may be sarcastic and make jokes about their problems. After ventilation, they may be able to talk about their frustrations with their current situation.[10] The nurse may be able to assist directly with the problems or may need to direct patients and families to appropriate resources. The results of emotional expression include the healing of sadness, the relief of fear, and the release of anger.

Everyone has built-in protective mechanisms that block painful emotions. These mechanisms are defenses that are activated automatically and unconsciously by the mind.[11] They are gradually lowered as the patient and family release emotions and adapt to their situation.[12]

Communication Safety Alert

To be effective as a nurse, you must understand and accept the emotions of patients and families, no matter what, to create an atmosphere of safety and trust. Understanding and acceptance do not mean that you have to agree with the patient. Patients do the best they can, given their circumstances at the time.

Empathy Versus Sympathy in Nurse-Patient Relationships

An important patient-safe communication strategy to use in managing emotional responses of patients, and in transforming negative communication climates to positive ones, is empathy. When you demonstrate empathy, you participate in the life of another and perceive that person's thoughts or feelings. It means putting yourself in the patient's place and seeing the human side of the patient. It also means being sensitive to the patient's private world. Once you have perceived the emotional response, you must respond to feelings and values in the situation and arrive at what is really important to the person. You must show you have sensitivity to the situation by communicating carefully with verbal and nonverbal behaviors to demonstrate that sensitivity. The result of empathy is that the person feels really understood. You have created common meaning and established a postive communication climate.[10,13,14]

Empathy also means that you remain emotionally separate from the other person, even though you can understand the patient's viewpoint. This is different from sympathy. Sympathy implies taking on the other's needs and problems as if they were your own and becoming emotionally involved to the point of losing your objectivity.[15]

Communication Safety Alert

To empathize rather than sympathize, you must show feelings but not get caught up in feelings or overly identify with the patient's and family's concerns. You will lose your objectivity if you share feelings so closely with a patient or family that your ability to think clearly and analyze problems becomes blocked.

Using the Patient-Safe Strategy of Empathy

The objective of using the patient-safe strategy of empathy is to convey interest in and understanding of the concerns behind painful emotions. You must listen long enough to allow the other person to experience release. You function as a sounding board and personal confidant.

First, through empathy, you convey that the patient is not alone and that you will be there to help the patient through the situation. You will then act as a patient advocate to help the patient and family in doing whatever it takes to make sure their health-care needs are met.[14,16]

Second, you should make it clear that there may be some things that the patient has not thought about that can be used to help handle the problem in a meaningful way. At this point, you become an educational resource, helping the patient and family to think critically and analyze the situation. If a patient or family member can identify some areas that can be controlled, self-esteem will most likely increase, and the underlying emotional distress will probably decrease.

❖ THE NURSE'S EMOTIONS

Emotions can be contagious, and you may feel the same emotions and tensions the patient and family feel. You may feel in danger of losing emotional control, and you may not know what to say or do. Acknowledge and accept emotions in yourself as well as your patient. Do not try to pretend that your emotions or your patients' emotions do not exist. They must not be ignored. They are present, real, and human. You must be aware of your emotions and how they are affecting the communication climate in nurse-patient relationships. Your emotions may lead to creation of negative or positive communication climates between you and the patient and influence communication outcomes.

Communication Safety Alert

Withholding your own emotional response leaves patients feeling out of control, unacceptable, and maybe even wondering if they are mentally unbalanced or crazy to feel the way they feel. You must carefully respond to patients, both verbally and nonverbally, using all of the listening responses and especially empathy.

Nursing students must learn to control their nervousness in patient care situations. Remember, emotions are transmitted back and forth between people and lead to positive or negative communication climates. You will be transmitting your anxieties to the patient, which will make the patient nervous.

Communication Safety Alert

If you are very nervous, there is no way that you can focus on the patient's emotions, because all you can concentrate on is the procedure and your own feelings about it. As you become calm and confident in doing technical procedures, you will be better able to focus on the patient's emotional state and manage the communication climate.

Managing Our Own Emotions

Individuals can learn to control their emotional response to situations. We can choose to respond in a different manner than what we have previously learned. There are two key reasons for developing skill in managing your emotions. First, managing emotions will improve your health. Research reveals that individuals who suppress or deny their emotions may develop a host of ailments such as cancer, asthma, heart disease, and increased blood pressure.[17] Second, managing emotions will improve your personal and professional relationships.[18]

Principles for Managing Emotions

The following are some principles that will help you to manage your emotions.

Recognize your feelings: It is important not to deny your feelings. When asked the question, "How do you feel?" we have a tendency to answer with a fact or a thought and not actually how we feel. Many people have difficulty expressing how they feel.[19] Expressing feelings may be associated with character weakness, may create an undesired sense of vulnerability, or may create a fear of rejection. Become attuned to your physiological responses that tell you how you are feeling. An increased heart rate, sweaty palms, and losing concentration are all signs of adrenaline release that accompany a highly emotional state. Monitor your nonverbal behavior, and recognize the feelings associated with raising your voice, waving your hands as you speak, and moving closer to or further away from the person with whom you speak. These are key signs for helping you connect with your emotional state.

Cool off: When your emotions manifest physiologically, in particular emotions such as shame and anger, it is best to allow for a cooling-off period. Otherwise, you may say something that you will soon regret and damage the relationship. Remember that communication is irreversible. You must learn to recognize your typical style of behavior when you become upset, and you must learn to control these behaviors when you are in a professional relationship.[20]

Take responsibility for your feelings: People do not make you feel emotions; you create these emotional responses by how you perceive and assign meaning to messages and life events. Albert Ellis describes how we own our feelings and have control over our emotions.[21] Consider a situation where you were called names. In one situation, the name calling came from a friend, and in another it came from someone who was intoxicated. The name calling from a friend could lead you to believe and assign meaning that you had done something wrong. The emotional feelings associated with this thought could be hurt, guilt, shame, or worry. The name calling from someone intoxicated would lead you to believe and assign meaning based on your interpretations that the individual is cognitively impaired. The feeling associated with this thought may be pity or amusement. In both situations, the same event occurred: you were called names. But your feelings arising from your interpretations and assigned meaning differed. The point to be made is that you create your own emotional responses; no one does this for you.

Owning Your Emotions: Use of "I" Statements

The communication strategy for owning your emotions is to use "I" language. An "I statement" begins with the word "I." The strategy was developed in the 1970s by Thomas Gordon.[22] Taking responsibility for your emotions says a great deal about you and influences the trust established within interpersonal and professional relationships. "I" language demonstrates assertiveness without putting the other communicator on the defensive. The use of "I" statements shows a willingness to accept responsibility for owning your thoughts and feelings. "I" statements typically involve three components[22]: your feelings, the behavior, and the consequences the behavior has on you.

Handling Emotions and Responding to a Personal Attack

We have a tendency to become emotionally distraught and respond defensively when people convey messages that personally attack us. Defensiveness is a means to protect ourselves from any challenge that threatens our sense of self-esteem and our ability to save face. There are two essential strategies to be used when under personal attack.[2]

The first strategy is to seek more information from the individual who is attacking you. You need to determine what the person is really saying or really feeling. For example, if you are accused with, "You are so rude," ask an open-ended clarifying question, "What do I do that is rude?" Focus on pulling the communication to a clarification of *behavior* and away from a personal attack. Often, the communicator will adopt a different tone by the mere fact that you are actively listening. Depending on the personal attack statement, you may be able to determine specifics by paraphrasing and using open-ended questions. The person says to you, "We are always late because of you. Have you no respect for being on time?" You reply, "It sounds like you are upset that I took so long to get ready. Am I right?" Again, try to remove the personal attack and uncover the underlying issue that is causing the problem.

The second strategy is to determine if there are some aspects of the criticism with which you can agree.[2] Often, we can find some truth in criticism. For example, "You are right; I do take a long time to return messages." Criticisms that describe a specific behavior and provide an offensive evaluation of the behavior can be challenging to respond to non-defensively. It is the offensive evaluation component that we have a hard time dealing with.[2] The following is an example of a criticism with accompanying offensive evaluation: "There is much to organize and plan when you are trying to build a deck. *You are ridiculous* to think you could do it in one weekend." The truth is there is much to organize when building a deck. The offensive evaluation is that "you are ridiculous." To respond non-defensively, agree with the truth in the criticism only if it is correct, and do not accept the evaluation. Your response could be, "You are right. There is a lot to organize and plan for building a deck. But I don't think that I'm ridiculous." The focus should be on responding to the criticism of the behavior, instead of reacting to the offensive evaluation that is a personal attack.

CHAPTER SUMMARY

This chapter focused on the nature of communication climates created by individuals in relationships and how negative and positive communications develop in health-care settings. Specifically, nurses must be aware of the tone, emotions, and attitudes of all communicators, including themselves. The nurse must identify a patient's emotional response to the illness and use basic patient-safe communication strategies to help the patient express emotions and enhance the communication climate. The nurse must create an atmosphere in which the patient feels valued and an important part of the health-care team.

The chapter also described the need for you to develop an awareness of your own emotional responses in clinical situations and how they affect the communication climate. You must learn to manage your personal emotional responses to promote postive communication climates.

BUILDING HIGH-LEVEL COMMUNICATION COMPETENCY

For additional exercises, see DavisPlus at http://davisplus.fadavis.com

1. In an exercise called visual imagery, picture yourself in the most beautiful, relaxing location you can envision,[23] sitting on a beach in the warm sun, for example. Close your eyes and hear the waves splashing against the shore. Feel the warm sun on your skin. Feel the warm ocean breeze on your face. See the gulls gliding gracefully across the glistening water. Say to yourself, "I am relaxed, I am relaxed, I am relaxed." Just make sure the visual image has meaning to you. This is another good technique that can be used to help patients relax.

2. Practice using the basic patient-safe communication strategies described in this chapter to demonstrate empathy toward a classmate. Use active listening and empathy to encourage a classmate to express his or her ideas and feelings about an important life event. One student should tell the story of the important life event, and the other one should use empathic patient-safe communication strategies to listen fully and facilitate the expression of ideas and emotions. After the storyteller finishes, the listener should summarize his or her perception of the content and feelings expressed to validate the storyteller's message. The storyteller will then state whether the summary is accurate.

References

1. Allen, W., Shea, J. Know Yourself and the Communication Climate. Located at http://www.allenshea.com/knowyourself.html Accessed November, 2008.
2. Adler, R.B., Rosenfeld, L.B., Proctor R.F., et al. Interplay: The Process of Interpersonal Communication. Don Mills, Ontario, Canada, Oxford University Press: 2006.
3. Burggraf, C.S., Sillars, A.L. A Critical Examination of Sex Differences in Marital Communication. Communication Monographs 54:276-294, 1987.

4. Cissna, K.N., Sieberg, E. Patterns of Interactional Confirmation and Disconfirmation. In Stewart, J. (ed.), Bridges, Not Walls, 7th ed. N.Y., McGraw-Hill: 1999, pp 336-346.

5. Beebe, S.A., Beebe, S.J., Redmond, M.V., et al. Interpersonal Communication: Relating to Others, 4th ed. Toronto, Ontario, Canada: Pearson Education Canada, 2007.

6. Festinger, L.A. A Theory of Cognitive Dissonance. Stanford, Calif., Stanford University Press: 1957.

7. Martin, H., Prange, A. The Stages of Illness: Psychosocial Approach. Nursing Outlook 10:168, 1962.

8. Kübler-Ross, E: On Death and Dying. N.Y., Macmillan: 1969.

9a. Kübler-Ross, E., Kessler, D. On Grief and Grieving: Finding the Meaning of Grief Through the Five Stages. Riverside, N.J., Simon and Schuster: 2005.

9b. Parsons, T. The Social System. N.Y., Free Press: 1951.

10. Rogers, C.R. Client-Centered Therapy. N.Y., Houghton Mifflin: 1951.

11. Freud, S. Complete Psychological Works: London, Hogarth Press: 1964.

12. Zook, R. Learning to Use Positive Defense Mechanisms. American Journal of Nursing 98:16B, 1998.

13. Sutherland, J.A. Historical Concept Analysis of Empathy. Issues in Mental Health Nursing 16:555, 1995.

14. Hoiat, M. Empathy in Patient Care: Antecedents, Development, Measurement, and Outcomes. N.Y., Springer: 2007.

15. Sundeen, S.J. Nurse-Client Interaction: Implementing the Nursing Process, 5th ed. St. Louis, Mosby: 1994.

16. Berman, A.J., Snyder, S.J., Kozier, B.J., et al. Kozier & Erb's Fundamentals of Nursing: Concepts, Process and Practice, 8th ed. Upper Saddle River, N.J., Prentice Hall: 2008.

17. Mayne, T.J.: Negative Affect and Health: The Importance of Being Earnest. Cognition and Emotion 13:601-635, 1999.

18. Kennedy-Moore, E., Watson, J.C. Expressing Emotion: Myths, Realities, and Therapeutic Strategies. N.Y., Guilford Press: 1999.

19. Peper, M. Awareness of Emotions: A Neuropsychological Perspective. In Ellis, R.D., Newton, N. (eds.), The Caldron of Consciousness: Motivation, affect and Self-Organization—An Anthology. Philadelphia, John Benjamins: 2000, pp 243-269.

20. American Psychological Association. Controlling Anger Before It Controls You. Located at www.apa.org/topics/controlanger.html Accessed October, 2009.

21. Ellis, A. Overcoming Destructive Beliefs, Feeling, and Behaving: New Directions for Rational Emotive Behavior Therapy. Amherst, N.Y., Prometheus Books: 2001.

22. Gordon, T. TET: Teacher Effectiveness Training. N.Y., Wyden: 1974.

23. Samuels, M., Samuels, N. Seeing With the Mind's Eye. N.Y., Random House: 1975.

The Patient-Safe Communication Strategy of Touch

Learning Outcomes

Upon completion of this chapter, you will be able to:

1. Identify why touch is a basic form of human communication.
2. Describe the basic human need for touch throughout life.
3. Identify the three basic forms of touch used by nurses as patient-safe communication strategies.
4. Describe the cultural implications of touch.
5. Integrate proxemics in nurse-patient relationships.
6. Identify appropriate nursing behaviors in each zone of personal space.
7. Distinguish between situations when touch is and is not appropriate.
8. Describe the physiological and psychological benefits of touch.

Key Words

Caring touch
Task touch
Protective touch

The primary purpose of this chapter is to help you develop an understanding of touch and its effective use in nursing practice as a patient-safe communication strategy. Examine the transformational model in Chapter 2, and locate touch in the patient-safe communication strategies ring. Touch is used as an instrument of patient safety because it can help to overcome and reduce many risk factors that block creation of common meaning and positive transformational outcomes. Appropriate use of touch requires high-level communication competency and is a critical and indispensible patient-safe communication strategy when administering nursing care.[1,2] *For an interactive version of this activity, see DavisPlus at http://davisplus.com.*[3] In doing the self-assessment, you can determine your current motivation to touch based on your past experiences. Do not worry if you score below average; this chapter will help you understand how to practice touch in an appropriate manner and how to use touch as a patient-safe communication strategy.

TOUCH IN GENERAL

Nursing has always been a very "high-touch" profession. Nurses provide hands-on care when patients are not able to care for themselves. These activities include: bathing, feeding, moving from bed to chair, assisting with walking, and other personal care for patients in addition to physical assessments and treatments. Nurses must learn how and when to touch as well as when not to touch. Touch is the most basic form of human nonverbal communication. Through touch, humans communicate such emotions as love, anger, and fear. In childhood, we see the raw forms of emotional expression through touch such as hitting, biting, pinching, hugging, and kissing. As adults, we learn through socialization to control the way we touch to express our emotions.

As with any communication strategy, some of us are better at using and interpreting touches than others. The way you have learned to touch other humans is, in part, the result of your life experiences and cultural influences.[4] Research has shown, for instance, that children of "high-touch" families are touchers as adults.[5,6] People of Italian, Jewish, Spanish, and South American ethnic backgrounds report touching more frequently than those of German and British ancestry. To research public displays of touch between different cultures, Sidney Jourard counted the number of touches per hour among couples sitting in cafes in various countries. He found 180 touches per hour in Puerto Rico, 110 touches per hour in Paris, 2 touches per hour in Gainesville, Florida, and 0 touches per hour in London.[7] These findings illustrate the influence of culture on touch.

In general, North Americans are very careful about whom they touch. Reasons for this reticence include the fear that a touch may be misinterpreted as having sexual overtones or be perceived as controlling.[8] People worry about accusations of sexual harassment and abuse in schools and workplaces. A slogan of the National Education Association, whose membership includes millions of teachers, sums up the perspective in North America today: "Teach, don't touch." While the slogan is certainly too broad in scope to become the rule for teachers, it is understandable why the organization believes it has to protect its members by emphasizing not touching. Alternately, research has indicated that waitresses who touched customers on the shoulder or hand as they returned change received bigger tips than those who did not.[9]

🧩 PATIENT-SAFE TOUCHING IN NURSING TAKES PRACTICE

Nurses use three basic forms of touch, sometimes touching patients in very intimate ways.[10-12] First, nurses use *emotionally supportive*, *caring touches* to help patients express themselves, to comfort patients during emotional distress, to show patients that they are valued and respected, and to gain their cooperation. Second, nurses use *procedural task touches* to perform technical care. For example, you can significantly decrease the pain of an injection by pressing the site with your thumb, hard enough to feel resistance, and maintaining the pressure for 10 seconds.[13] Third, nurses use *protective touches* to keep patients from harming themselves or others. For example, a cognitively impaired patient will be restrained when on a ventilator to prevent him from pulling out the tubes.

Communication Safety Alert

Whether using caring, procedural, or protective touches, nurses use touch as a patient-safe communication strategy to promote positive health-care outcomes and positive transformations.

Most beginning nursing students are anxious about touching patients.[14] They are awkward and embarrassed about viewing and touching typically unexposed "private parts" of human anatomy and touching patients in intimate areas. For example, in fundamentals courses, students typically are hesitant and anxious about performing basic procedures, such as a bed bath. When learning health assessment, a male student may wonder in embarrassment what he is supposed to do with a woman's breast while he tries to find her apical pulse.

Some students feel awkward even when performing touch in seemingly innocuous situations, such as picking up a patient's arm to put on a blood pressure cuff. Many students lack knowledge and self-confidence in how to touch patients who are emotionally distressed, in pain, anxious, or agitated. Keep in mind that touch is like any other nursing skill. Anxiety and awkwardness are typical, natural reactions whenever learning and performing something new. As you gain practice in touching patients, you will become much more comfortable doing so and you also will develop your own professional patient-safe touching style.

🧩 TOUCH: A BASIC HUMAN NEED

Touch is a basic human need, as necessary for survival as food, clothing, and shelter.[15] It is the first sense to develop in humans and remains until death. In 1248, German emperor Frederick II was curious to see what language children would speak if no one talked to them or cuddled them. He conducted his "research" by taking newborns from their parents and having "nurses" feed them without talking to them or cuddling them. The babies all died before speaking because of the lack of touch.[9]

It is important to recognize your own cultural beliefs about the importance of touch. For example, suppose that you have fed and changed a 6-month-old baby and you put her in her crib for a nap. You have done everything you can think of to prepare the baby for her nap, and she is not sick in any way. But the baby starts to cry when you lay her down. Would your mother and family tell you to hold and rock the baby, to let the baby cry to exercise her lungs, or to ignore the crying to avoid spoiling the baby? At present, child authorities generally advise picking up a baby when it cries to meet the baby's security needs and ultimately affect the development of a baby's self-concept. In other words, the baby learns to trust others and that he or she is important, resulting in a positive self-concept.[8] Touch provides infants with security necessary for normal psychological development.[16,17]

Touch has been found to be beneficial for humans in many ways. Studies of massage in premature infants have shown that a 15-minute massage three times daily led to hospital discharge 6 days early, at a savings of $10,000 per infant.[18,19] Other studies have shown that handling increases visual alertness in babies and also has soothing effects.[17,20]

Touch also supplies the security needed for exploration as a toddler. Children explore their environment and repeatedly run back to their mothers for reassurance. After consolation, they feel secure to return to their exploration.

Does it follow that, as people grow into adults, they still need touch? Hollender conducted interviews of men and women to determine the adult desire to hold or be held.[21,22] Most people indicated a moderate desire to be held, with men nearly as high as women in their ratings of the desire to hold or to be held. He found that many adults reported an increased need for touch when they were depressed or anxious. Touch has been described as the ultimate intimacy in humans.[23] Although the need for touch does not go away in adulthood, the need may be neglected or ignored, resulting in lonliness and depression.

The Physiological Response of the Body to Touch

Nurses must have a thorough understanding of the physiological response of the body to touch. Touch can be used to decrease a patient's response to stress.[24] Whenever a person feels apprehension and pain, the body launches a stress response, a sequence of biochemical events. The perception of stress by the cortex and hypothalamus of the brain activates the interactive autonomic nervous system, the psychoneuroendocrine system, and the musculoskeletal system.[25] A well-known effect of stress is increased muscular tension and rigidity. Motor pathways of the autonomic nervous system stimulate the musculoskeletal system, along with stimulation by hormones from the psychoneuroendocrine system.

Touch transmits messages to the brain to calm the stress response. The skin contains millions of touch receptors—up to 3000 in just a fingertip—that send messages along the spinal cord to the brain. Once these messages arrive, the brain regulates the autonomic and psychoneuroendocrine systems. The body produces endorphins, which are the body's natural way of suppressing pain. Also, production of cortisol and norepinephrine decreases. Cortisol suppresses immune functioning, and norepinephrine prepares for the fight-or-flight response by increasing heart rate, blood pressure, and breathing.

It is clear that touch has physiogical ramifications. A simple, caring touch to a shoulder or the feel of an arm around a waist can reduce the heart rate and lower blood pressure. That is why a mother hugging a child with a skinned knee may actually make the child better from a physiological standpoint. Touch, when administered effectively, can stimulate positive physiological responses in the body.

NURSES USE TOUCH

Nurses have social permission to touch people. The social permission cuts across all cultures. In other words, patients expect nurses to touch them. Social permission means that people will allow and actually expect nurses to touch them during procedures. They also allow and expect nurses to provide comforting touches. Touching is part of the nurse's job description. Beginning nursing student typically wonder if patients will allow them to perform procedures or give comforting touches. Research on touch and male nursing students has shown men to be especially concerned that their comfort touches may be misinterpreted as flirtatious or sexual.[26] Male and female students need reassurance that touch in the nurse-patient relationship is expected and welcome. Most people like to be touched. Most patients willingly accept and welcome touches from nurses and nursing students.

Intent of Touch

The primary factor that determines how a patient will respond to touch is the intention of the touch. Jones suggests that touch needs to be related to the context of the situation.[8] The meaning of the touch relates to the situation, the timing, and the manner in which the touch is delivered.

Communication Safety Alert

You will need to evaluate each situation carefully and then deliver appropriate touches. Thus, a hand on a patient's shoulder can convey, "I want to comfort you," "I like you," or "I was just kidding."

You need to become familiar with the three basic intents of touch that have been identified in nursing: caring touch, task touch, and protective touch. You also need to know when it is appropriate to use and not to use touch.[10-12]

Caring Touch

Caring touch has an emotional intent and involves comforting touch and encouraging touch. Comforting touch includes holding a patient's hand, stroking the forehead, squeezing the shoulder, stroking the arm, and placing a hand on the chest. These types of touch are usually associated with dying, discomfort, or grief. Specifically, patients who are in pain, anxious, frightened, confused, or agitated often respond very positively to touch. They will openly express their appreciation and reciprocate the touch. For example, consider the family member who reported that his wife's favorite nurse spent a few minutes each day holding her hand and stroking her forehead when she was very ill during chemotherapy for breast cancer. He described her as the "best nurse" because of how much she cared about his wife as a person.

Encouraging touches include placing an arm around the shoulders, giving a hug or a pat on the back, and playful hitting and poking. Encouraging touch is more hopeful and future-oriented and is often used to celebrate clinical progress. These touches are used for supporting, reassuring, and raising the spirits of patients and families. For example, several hours after nursing a patient through a difficult labor, a labor and delivery nurse visits a patient and asks how she is doing and immediately gives her a hug. The hug conveys congratulations and also emotional support at that special time. Research indicates that hand holding before anesthesia usually makes the procedure less frightening.[27] Also during surgery, a nurse may stand at the foot of the bed and lay a hand on the foot or ankle of the patient or may stand at the head of the bed and lay a hand on the patient's face to reduce the patient's anxiety.[27]

Task Touch

Most touch in nursing is task touch, which involves physical assessment and procedural treatments that must be done. Gender differences in touch have been the focus of studies. Characteristically, men are less gentle when touching others than women are.[28,29] The objective is to be as gentle, soft, and careful with task touches as you can be. Task touch should overlap with caring touch. Through gentle, soft, and careful touch during assessments and procedures, you will communicate warmly that you value and respect patients and that you really do care about them. In contrast, hurried, rough, jarring touches communicate coldness and that you do not value and respect the patient.

Protective Touch

Physically protective touches for patients involve exerting control over the patient in a situation in which patient safety is a primary concern. It is best to combine protective touch with caring touch whenever possible. For example, patients sometimes need to be held down to keep them from harming themselves. Confused patients may be restrained and sedated to ensure that they will not pull on vital tubes or fall out of a bed or chair. It is often helpful to use caring touch with a patient who is being restrained. The patient's hand can be gently held down as someone else carefully applies the restraint.

Take care, though, to minimize the danger of being hurt by a combative patient who may attempt to strike or harm you. Say, for example, that an elderly woman who had gallbladder surgery has a reaction to the anesthetic. She becomes disoriented, does not know where she is, and attempts to pull out her intravenous line and get out of bed. She is very strong, and it takes two male attendants to hold her down while you gently apply restraints. The next morning, when the anesthetic has worn off and she is fully alert, you can safely remove the restraints.

Inhibition of Nursing Touch

The lack of touch and the use of task touch without adding caring touches have been described as emotionally protective to the nurse. Nursing research suggests that nurses who are task-oriented may be distancing themselves from pain and suffering as a means of protecting themselves emotionally.[10,11] The nurse may feel a loss of concern for the patient and family.[30] The burned-out nurse has little or no emotional energy to relate to patients. In general, the better the nurse feels physically and emotionally, the greater the ability to relate to patients by touch or any other patient-safe communication strategy.

Harsh or severe touches have been related to tension being released by the nurse. Nurses and other health-care providers who are unable to communicate effectively, either verbally or nonverbally with confused and agitated patients, become frustrated. Frustration leads to tension, and tension must be released. Nurses may have feelings of reaching the "end of their rope" and quickly move to sedate and restrain patients, using harsh touches that release their own emotional tension.[11]

In addition, research indicates that some patient characteristics decrease the amount of caring touches administered to them.[11] For example, patients with behavioral problems—such as those who are demanding, verbally abusive, and uncooperative—receive less caring touch and more protective touch. Those with contagious diseases, such as acquired immunodeficiency syndrome (AIDS) or tuberculosis, may receive fewer touches if the nurse fears acquiring the disease. Also, patients perceived as responsible for their own conditions, such as alcoholics or drug addicts who repeatedly overdose, typically receive less touch.[11] It is unfortunate that these patients receive less touch because they are the ones most in need of caring touch and other forms of emotional support.

GETTING STARTED WITH PATIENT-SAFE TOUCH

The best way to find out if a patient is receptive to touch is to try it. Begin with a handshake when you first meet your patient. Watch the patient's reaction carefully. Look for grimacing or body tensing. Note whether the patient pulls away, lets a hand linger, or perhaps clings to your hand.

If you care for that patient on a second day, again offer a handshake and to show warmth and respect. One student reported that an elderly woman patient was so starved for touch that the patient pulled her down into the bed to give her a hug. Providing comforting touches to elderly patients often improves feelings of well-being in both the elderly and the health professional.[31,32]

Shaking Hands

Handshaking has become a means of communicating how people feel about each other. We have all experienced the variations of handshakes, including differences in pressure, duration, and awkwardness. Chances are that you already understand the rules of the customary handshake in Western civilizations. A hearty, firm grip is supposed to indicate that you are sincere and pleased to meet someone. Men usually have a stronger handshake grip than women.[28,29]

Look the person directly in the eyes and smile during the handshake. Verbal expressions that are used with the handshake include, "Glad to meet you" and "How are you today?" Some people respond by grasping the elbow or forearm of the other person's arm. A few grasp the extended hand with both hands and shake. Both variations indicate extra affection and friendliness.[9]

In general, handshakes are required as you meet someone for the first time, whether you introduce yourself or are introduced by someone else. In the past, men alone shook hands, not women. Today women are expected to shake hands when they are introduced to each other or to men. As you introduce yourself to your patient and family for the first time, you may greet them with a handshake.

Suppose you have just met your patient for the day, shaken hands, and noted that the patient held on to your hand for a few seconds longer than you would have otherwise expected. She smiled at you as you shook her hand. Both the lingering hand and the smile lets you know she responded to your touch positively.

Next, you plan to do a brief physical assessment to be sure she is progressing physically as expected, and then you want to discuss plans for how to proceed with the tasks that need to be done that day. You begin by pulling back the sheets and lifting her gown. The patient frowns, clings to her covers, and says, "What are you going to do to me?" What went wrong?

Entering Personal Space

You violated rules for entering personal space by pulling back her covers without asking permission and without letting her know what you were going to do before you did it. You need to be very aware of personal space and the rules that apply when moving about within the personal space of each individual. Proxemics involves the study of personal space and the meaning of proximity or closeness of one person to another as the distance between the two people increases or decreases.[33]

The Intimate Zone

The intimate zone of personal space is from the skin surface to about 16 inches away from the body. This is the zone violated when the covers were drawn back without warning. People guard this zone the most. This zone is reserved for close friends and relatives, for those with whom there is emotional closeness. Nurses and other health-care providers must ask permission to enter this zone.

Tell a person what you are going to do before you attempt to do it. Explain sensations that the patient can expect to feel as you touch so that the patient will not think anything out of the ordinary is being experienced. Explaining the steps and sensations in a procedure as you go along guides the patient and decreases anxiety.

Communication Safety Alert

Warm your hands and your stethoscope before touching the patient. Few things make someone tense and withdraw faster than cold hands. Use slow, deliberate, gentle, and purposeful touches as you do your assessment or any procedure, watching the patient's nonverbal responses. Always ask permission, and let the patient know what you will be doing before you touch, even for the simplest procedure, such as a blood pressure.

The Personal Zone

A bit further out, from 1.5 to 4 feet, is the personal zone. This is generally the zone that is used most often, especially for socializing. People typically stand this far apart at parties and friendly gatherings. In nursing, this is the zone in which to conduct a personal history and to discuss plans for how to proceed with the activities that must be done on any given day. Sit at the same height as the patient, and discuss the plan and options quietly. If the patient sits and you stand, you create a position of dominance and give the impression of not having much time to sit and discuss the plan of care. If you want to find out if the patient is having any problems or feeling any discomfort, you need to move to within 4 feet and get on the same level as the patient.

Communication Safety Alert

Beginning students need to get accustomed to being in the personal zone with a person who would otherwise be a stranger. Typically, you would not stand so close to a stranger. There is a set of expectations about how you should act in the role of nurse. One of these expectations is that you are within personal distance most of the time, especially if you want to develop effective nurse-patient relationships and encourage patients to respond to you as you would like them to.

The Social Zone

From 4 to 12 feet away from a person is the social zone. This is an impersonal zone, and it is the space used for strangers and for people we do not know. This zone is often misused in nursing. Most of what is done in nursing requires the use of the personal zone because what is discussed is private.

Communication Safety Alert

When you stand in the social zone to discuss personal matters, you give the impression of being impersonal and not caring. For example, imagine a nurse who stands in the doorway of a semiprivate room and announces to Mrs. Jones in bed A that it is time for her enema. Mrs. Jones would much rather have kept her bowel status personal and would be embarrassed by the announcement and probably upset with the nurse for being insensitive. The nurse should have used the personal zone.

The Public Zone

Distances that exceed 12 feet from a person are in the public zone. A person giving a speech would stand at least 12 feet from the audience. You might use the public zone during patient educational activities that involve giving a lecture to a group of patients and their families.

Cultural Dictates

The preceding generalizations about personal space are based on research involving European North Americans. The distances in the four zones are averages that have been computed based on observations of North Americans. Keep in mind that different cultures draw different lines around personal space. So, depending on your ethnic background, you or your patient may need more or less personal space.

For example, descendants of Hispanics, Middle Easterners, and southern Europeans (Italians, French, Spanish, and so on) stand much closer to each other and feel comfortable. Descendants from Asia and Northern Europe (Germany, England, Ireland, and so on) may not feel as comfortable in proximity because they are used to having more space.

As you keep these zones and the behaviors expected within them in mind, temper that knowledge with the fact that you must allow the patient and family to select the distance that is comfortable to them when they are talking to you.

Painful Touches

One rule that transcends all cultures is never inflict pain on another through touch, even accidentally.[8] Some nursing procedures are uncomfortable, and some hurt. Many students feel bad about purposefully performing such procedures as dressing changes, suture removal, injections, and catheterizations. You must learn the correct way to perform each procedure so that it produces the least amount of pain, and you must use pain medication appropriately before such procedures.

Communication Safety Alert

During painful procedures, talk gently, and coach the patient. Avoid giving patients the impression that they are objects to be worked on. If a procedure requires your full attention, a second person should be available strictly for emotional support and coaching the patient throughout the procedure. Apologize during and after the procedure, "I know this hurts, but I will be done in a minute. Thank you for holding still." Afterward, "I'm sorry I hurt you. You were very patient and cooperative."

Hugging

Nurses can learn to give compassionate and supportive hugs that are thoughtful and respectful. Hugs can be therapeutic when the intention is to show that you care and want to comfort a patient or family member of the patient.[34] Hugging a child before the induction of anesthesia may make it less frightening, for example.

As you read this, you might be thinking, "What about the sexual overtones of a hug?" Hugs that nurses dispense are compassionate, not passionate. Patients recognize the difference.

Communication Safety Alert

Be certain that you have permission before hugging. A hug is within the intimate zone and, therefore, requires permission. Sometimes the permission may be nonverbal, and you respond spontaneously. Or you could ask, "Can I give you a hug?"

There are many types of hugs for different purposes. You will develop your own hugging style and a sense for when a hug is needed and acceptable. Keating, in her book on hug therapy, described 10 types of hugs.[35] Three hugs that are especially useful in nursing situations are the A-frame hug, the side-to-side hug, and the bear hug,

A-Frame Hug
This involves wrapping two arms around the shoulders of the patient and leaning in toward the patient until your shoulders and cheeks touch. This hug is brief, and nothing below the shoulders makes contact. Patients may also wrap their arms around your shoulders. If you have not had much experience hugging, this is a comfortable and nonthreatening hug to try first. This hug is classic and formal, and it can be used with new acquaintances or professional colleagues. It is often used in some cultures as a hello or goodbye hug and may be combined with a kiss on the cheek.

Side-to-Side Hug
This is a one-armed squeeze around the shoulder or the waist of another. It is a more playful hug. Suppose you are walking with a patient, supporting her around the shoulders or waist. As you help her back into bed, you might give her a squeeze and tell her what a good job she did walking and that she is making good progress. If the patient is crying or frightened, you may gently put an arm around her shoulders or waist to offer emotional support.

Bear Hug
This involves bodies touching in a powerful, strong squeeze that can last for 5 to 10 seconds and generate a warm, supportive, secure feeling. Take care to make the hug firm and not breathless, remembering always to be considerate of your partner. Parents share these hugs with children, giving a "You are terrific" message. Friends might give these hugs as a way to share joy or sorrow.

Communication Safety Alert

A patient with a history of abuse, either physical or sexual, may prefer little or no touch beyond what is needed to carry out tasks. Psychiatric patients may require special care with touch. Some patients will keep their distance and pull away to avoid a touch.

Nurses must become very sensitive to patients who withdraw from touch. If a patient withdraws as you touch, and you realize that you made a touch mistake, offer a brief apology such as, "I'm sorry, I did not mean to startle you." Your apology shows that you care and that you are aware of what happened.

Many students are concerned that patients may misinterpret their touches, even during a procedure. For example, young female students just learning to do bed baths commonly express concern about male patients becoming sexually stimulated during cleaning of the genitals. Likewise, male students express the same concerns as they learn to bathe females.[26] Avoid long, lingering touches anywhere, especially in private areas. In addition, remember that the majority of patients unable to perform their own perineal care are too sick to become aroused. As you clean, focus on the idea that perineal care is essential to prevent urinary tract infections.

Massage: A Classic Touch Technique

Massage has been promoted as providing benefits to mind, body, and spirit.[36] Massage techniques date back to ancient times, when Roman and Greek physicians used massage to alleviate pain, promote healing, and to relax and tone muscles. At present, massage is very popular as a means of reducing stress and helping with relaxation. Millions of Americans visit massage therapists yearly, and parents are learning how to give massages to their babies. Massages are even being offered at airports and shopping malls.

The medical research on massage is mounting, indicating that it has positive effects in many conditions, such as lowering anxiety in depressed adolescents, reducing agitation in Alzheimer's patients, easing stiffness and pain in arthritis sufferers, helping people with asthma breathe easier, and boosting immune functioning in AIDS patients.[9,35]

Nurses have traditionally given back massages as part of the morning bath procedure to stimulate circulation and reduce backaches in patients confined to bed. Back massages are also helpful in inducing relaxation when performed as part of the evening preparation for sleep. As described in many fundamental nursing texts, nurses learn to use a combination of techniques, including stroking, friction, pressure, and kneading for back massages. Many patients have opened up and talked about what is worrying them during or after a back massage. Although back rubs are not for everyone, many patients appreciate them and feel more secure following massages, believing that the nurse can be trusted and is interested in them.

You may be interested in integrating many other forms of touch therapies into your practice. Examples of touch therapies include acupuncture, acupressure, reflexology, and therapeutic touch. These therapies are not usually included in basic nursing education programs. Nurses require special certification courses before trying these therapies on patients.

CHAPTER SUMMARY

Nursing has a long history of employing touch to comfort and treat patients. Research indicates that touch as a patient-safe communication strategy can create a warm and caring atmosphere. Touch, a therapeutic patient-safe communication strategy that involves knowledge of how and how *not* to touch, takes much practice. Touch involves personal sensitivity to patients and health-care situations. As with any other patient-safe communication strategies, carefully monitor the patient's response to your touches, and use these responses to guide further communications.

HIGH-LEVEL COMPETENCY COMMUNICATION EXERCISES

For additional exercises, visit davisplus at http://davisplus.fadavis.com

1. Go up to someone you do not know in class, shake hands, and introduce yourself. Follow this up with a group discussion of the various ways that students in class shook hands and what this means based on past experiences.

2. Give the partner you just met a hug. Experiment exchanging the A-frame, side-to-side, and bear hugs with classmates. Follow the hugging with a group discussion of the type of hugs that were given in class and what this means based on your past experiences.

References

1. Gatlon, G. (ed.). Touch Papers: Dialogues on Touch in the Psychoanalytic Space. Karnac, London: 2006.
2. Chang, S.O. The Conceptual Structure of Physical Touch in Caring. Journal of Advanced Nursing 33:820-827, 2008.
3. Anderson, P.A., Leibowitz, K. The Development and Nature of the Construct Touch Avoidance. Environmental Psychology and Nonverbal Behavior 3:89, 1978.
4. Halley, J.O. Boundaries of Touch: Parenting and Adult-Child Intimacy. Urbana, Ill., University of Illinois Press, 2007.
5. Jones, S.E., Yarbrough, A.E. A Naturalistic Study of the Meanings of Touch. Communication Monograph 52:19, 1985.
6. Gladney, K., Barker, L. The Effects of Tactile History on Attitudes Toward and Frequency of Touching Behavior. Sign Language Studies 24:231, 1979.
7. Jourard, S.M. An Exploratory Study of Body Accessibility. British Journal of Social and Clinical Psychology 5:221, 1966.
8. Jones, S.E. The Right Touch: Understanding and Using the Language of Physical Contact. Cresskill, N.J., Hampton Press: 1994.
9. Colt, G.H., Schatz, H., Hollister, A. The Magic of Touch. Life 8:54–61, 1997.
10. Talton, C.W. Touch—of All Kinds—Is Therapeutic. RN 2:61, 1995.
11. Estabrooks, C.A. Touch: A Nursing Strategy in the Intensive Care Unit. Heart and Lung 18:392, 1989.
12. Adomat, R., Killingworth, A. Care of the Critically Ill Patient: The Impact of Stress on the Use of Touch in Intensive Therapy Units. Journal of Advanced Nursing 19:912, 1994.
13. Barnhill B.J., Holbert, M.D., Jackson, N.M., et al. Using Pressure to Decrease the Pain of Intramuscular Injections. Journal of Pain and Symptom Management 12:52, 1996.
14. Rombalski, J.J. A Personal Journey in Understanding Physical Touch as a Nursing Intervention. Journal of Holistic Nursing 21:73-80, 2003.
15. Caplan, M. To touch Is to Live: The Need for Genuine Affection in an Impersonal World. Prescott, Ariz., Hohm Press: 2002.
16. Reite, M.L. Touch, Attachment, and Health: Is There a Relationship? In Brown, C.C. (ed.). The Many Facets of Touch. Johnson & Johnson Baby Products Co., 1984, p. 58.
17. White, B.L., Castle, P.W. Visual Exploratory Behavior Following Postnatal Handling of Human Infants. Perceptual and Motor Skills 18:497, 1964.
18. Field, T. Tactile/Kinesthetic Stimulation Effects on Preterm Neonates. Pediatrics 77:654, 1986.
19. Field, T. Alleviating Stress in Newborn Infants in the Intensive Care Unit. Stimulation and the Preterm Infant 17:1, 1990.
20. Harrison, L. Effects of Gentle Human Touch on Preterm Infants: Pilot Study Results. Neonatal Network 15:35, 1996.
21. Hollender, M.H. The Need or Wish to Be Held. Archives of General Psychiatry 22:445, 1970.
22. Hollender, M.H. Wish to Be Held and Wish to Hold in Men and Women. Archives of General Psychiatry 33:49, 1976.
23. Grader, R. The Cuddle Sutra: An Unabashed Celebration of the Ultimate Intimacy. Naperville, Ill., Sourcebooks Casablanca: 2007.

24. Nelson, D. From the Heart Through the Hands: The Power of Touch in Caregiving. Forres, Findhorn, England: 2001.
25. Wells-Federman, C.L. The Mind-Body Connection: The Psychophysiology of Many Traditional Nursing Interventions. Clinical Nurse Specialist 9:59, 1995.
26. Harding, T. Suspect Touch: A Problem for Men in Nursing. Nursing Journal 12: 28-34, 2008.
27. Tovar, M.K. Touch: The Beneficial Effects for the Surgical Patient. Association of Perioperative Registered Nurses Journal 49:1356, 1989.
28. Glass, L. He Says, She Says: Closing the Communication Gap Between the Sexes. Berkeley, N.Y.: 1993.
29. Glass, L. I Know What You're Thinking: Using the Four Codes of Reading People to Improve Your Life. Hoboken, John Wiley & Sons: 2003.
30. Freudenberger, H.J. Staff Burnout. Journal of Social Issues 30:159, 1974.
31. Edvardsson, J.D., Sandman, P., Rasmussen, B.H. Meanings of Giving Touch in the Care of Older Patients: Becoming a Valuable Person and Professional. Journal of Clinical Nursing, 12:601-609, 2003.
32. Newson, P. A Comforting Touch: Enhancing Residents' Wellbeing. Nursing and Residential Care 10:269-273, 2008.
33. Hall, E.T. The Hidden Dimension. Garden City, N.Y., Anchor Books/Doubleday: 1966.
34. Post, E. Etiquette: The Blue Book of Social Usage. N.Y., Funk & Wagnall: 1940.
35. Keating, K. The Hug Therapy Book. Center City, Minn., Hazelden: 1995.
36. Field, T. Massage Therapy Research. Edinburgh, N.Y., Elsevier-Churchill Livingstone: 2006.

The Patient-Safe Communication Strategy of Humor

Learning Outcomes

Upon completion of this chapter, you will be able to:

1. Define humor and laughter.
2. Describe the general purposes of humor and laughter.
3. Describe the benefits of humor in facilitating communication.
4. Distinguish between humor that is therapeutic and nontherapeutic.
5. Describe the physiological and psychological effects of humor.
6. Describe how patients use humor.
7. Identify the appropriate uses of humor by nurses in health-care settings.
8. Describe how humor can be used as a patient-safe communication strategy to facilitate nurse-patient relationships.

Key Words

Therapeutic humor
Nontherapeutic humor

Arousal phase
Relaxation phase

Humor and laughter are important patient-safe communication strategies that are linked to healing and a sense of well-being. They are also effective therapeutic mechanisms for releasing stress-related tensions. A sense of humor, including the ability to laugh with others and to laugh at oneself, has been associated with good health for centuries. For example, during the 18th century, there was a saying that "the arrival of a single clown has a more healthful impact on the health of a village than that of 20 asses laden with medication."[1] This same idea is reflected in the modern version of the expression, "Laughter is the best medicine."[2] *For an interactive version of this activity, see DavisPlus at http://davisplus.fadavis.com.* In doing the self-assessment, you can determine your current ability to laugh at life based on your past experiences.

During the late 1970s, Norman Cousins stimulated a scientific interest in the health professions regarding the benefits of humor and laughter during illness. His popular book, *Anatomy of an Illness*, described how 10 minutes of laughter rendered him free of pain for 2 hours. He said that humor aided his recovery from ankylosing spondylitis, an immune disorder that causes pain and inflammation of bones and joints.[3,4] Since then, nurses and other health-care researchers have been exploring the therapeutic effects of humor and are finding ways to integrate humor into patient care situations and with each other.[5-14]

Therapeutic humor in health-care situations can be used as a patient-safe communication strategy. Therapeutic humor has been defined as: "Any intervention that promotes health and wellness by stimulating a playful discovery, expression or appreciation of the absurdity or incongruity of life's situations. This intervention may enhance health or be used as a complementary treatment of illness to facilitate healing or coping, whether physical, emotional, cognitive, social or spiritual."[15]

Nursing education programs and health-care institutions expect nurses to take their jobs very seriously, and they do. Nevertheless, many nurses have realized how beneficial humor can be when it is used appropriately. Humor is not appropriate in every situation. It is a patient-safe strategy that needs to be used after careful assessment of the situation and only with knowledge of the emotional state of the patient.[14,16]

Therapeutic humor as a patient-safe strategy in nursing involves the purposeful use of humor to establish relationships by accelerating the development of trust; relieving anxiety and fear; releasing and defusing anger, hostility, and aggression; and improving patient education.[5-13,17-21] Humor is an important patient-safe communication strategy used to reduce risk factors that block creation of common meaning and positive transformational outcomes.

Research suggests that patients expect and appreciate a sense of humor in their nurses and that a sense of humor is regarded as an important characteristic of a good nurse.[5,9,11,13,14,16,21-25] Humor makes health-care providers more human to patients and reduces the distance between the nurse and the patient. Patient safety is enhanced because the nurse-patient relationship is established and maintained through the use of humor.

Humor is located in the patient-safe communication strategies ring of the transformational model in Chapter 2. Appropriate use of humor requires high-level communication competency. The primary purpose of this chapter is to explore the effects of humor and appropriate and inappropriate uses of humor in nurse-patient relationships.

✦ HUMOR IN NURSE-PATIENT RELATIONSHIPS

Humor used as a patient-safe strategy helps to build and maintain nurse-patient relationships. Humor is therapeutic when it is used to help reduce stressful health-care situations and put the patient at ease. Therapeutic humor is a form of verbal or nonverbal communication that is used as an adaptive and healthy coping mechanism for reducing stress levels in numerous situations.[15]

Humor has been generally defined as something that is or has the ability to be funny or amusing and results in smiling or laughter.[12,13,17-20] Humor encompasses a number of activities, such as joking, kidding, teasing, clowning, and mimicking. Much of the humor in health settings is spontaneous and specific to a situation. Nurses or patients make witty or humorous comments, which make others laugh, smile, or feel amused. It typically does not entail formal joke telling.[8,12,13,17-20]

People express personality through humor. As a characteristic of one's personality, some people have more of a sense of humor and look regularly for the lighter side of a problem, whereas others take things much more seriously.[26] Having a healthy and mature sense of humor means laughing at the imperfections in ourselves and laughing with others about the imperfect nature of typical daily situations.[26-28] In addition to laughing with others, a sense of humor involves knowing how to make others laugh.[9-11,23] Patients reveal their sense of humor by joking about their troubles with illness, health insurance, medical bills, diagnostic tests and surgeries, and the care they receive from nurses, doctors, and other health-care providers. Likewise, nurses joke about these same things as well as high workloads, high staff turnover rates, ever-increasing technology, and never-ending paperwork.

Nontherapeutic Humor

Humor is not appropriate when it takes place at the expense of individuals or groups and alienates them. Jokes that tease maliciously and belittle someone or a group are termed put-downs. Jokes can be contemptuous or sarcastic and thus aggressive and hostile expressions of dislike and disdain. Ethnic humor or jokes about gender differences can be offensive and indicate prejudice. These jokes are intended as insults to express superiority over someone else.[8,14,16]

People who use this type of humor may have low self-esteem and feel insecure. In cases of low self-esteem, people build themselves up by putting others down. Instead of reducing tension, laughing at someone is insensitive and creates more stressful emotional tension.[1,14] Nurses need to be very careful never to be insulting with humor; they need to laugh with, but not at, patients and their families.

Humor is not appropriate when a patient is very sick or emotionally distraught. If someone is very fearful, very anxious, very sad, or in great pain, humor will not be appreciated. All of the person's energy is needed to ward off the danger, and the comic effect is lost. The dangerous threat must be controlled before reference to the problem can be enjoyed through humor.[6,7,13,14,17-19] When a patient is in a crisis situation, humor results in disgust or horror. For example, consider the patient who was in the recovery room and breathing heavily. The nurse had just assessed his pulse, blood pressure, and ventilatory status and believed that his heavy breathing resulted from anxiety. She said, "Hey buddy, how about controlling that heavy breathing? I've got goose bumps!" The patient was so upset he later stated, "She was so uncaring. I couldn't breathe because it hurt so bad, and she was making jokes!"

What is hilarious to one person can be insulting and tasteless to another. This difference depends on biophysical, psychological, social, cultural, and spiritual states of being. You must first "know your audience" to understand the effect of specific types of humor. The criteria for determining the appropriateness of humor are in the Communication Safety Alert.

Communication Safety Alert

Criteria for Determining Appropriateness of Humor (Adapted from Pasquali, E.A. Learning to Laugh: Humor as Therapy. Journal of Psychosocial Nursing 28:31, 1990.)

Anxiety level: Humor is appropriate when patient anxiety is in the mild-to-moderate range and when humor can decrease patient anxiety. Humor is inappropriate when patient anxiety is in the severe-to-panic range and when it increases patient anxiety.

Coping style: Humor is appropriate when it helps a patient cope more effectively, facilitates learning, puts the situation in perspective, or decreases social distance and when patient cognitive and emotional status permit understanding of and response to humor. Humor is inappropriate when it leads to avoiding dealing with problematic situations, when it masks feelings or increases social distance, and when psychopathology interferes with understanding of or response to humor.

Humor style: Humor is appropriate when it conforms with the type of humor and humorist that the patient enjoys and when it laughs *with* people (i.e., laughs at what people do, not at who they are). Humor is inappropriate when it ignores patient humor style and when it laughs *at* people (other-deprecating humor.)

PHYSIOLOGICAL EFFECTS OF LAUGHTER AND HUMOR

Humor often results in smiling and laughter. In addition to helping people feel good, laughter can help individuals heal. Indeed, it can help to prevent them from getting sick in the first place. Why do people feel so good after laughing? The answer to that question requires an understanding of the physiological responses of the body during laughter.[30] There are two basic phases of response to laughter: arousal and relaxation.

Arousal Phase

During arousal, catecholamines (such as adrenaline) increase, which speeds up breathing, heart rate, and blood pressure. Depending on how intense the laughter, various groups of muscles contract. When people laugh so hard that they cry, the tears produced contain steroids and other toxins that accumulate under stress.[2,31] Thus, through secretion of tears, the body regains a healthier biochemical balance. In addition, the immune system is stimulated into helping the body fight disease.[16,32-36] A smile causes the zygomaticus major face muscle to contract, which stimulates the "master" thymus gland to secrete thymosin and produce T-cell lymphocytes.[37] These lymphocytes are primary components of the immune defense system, which helps people stay healthy and fight disease. Laughter also increases an antibody in saliva that prevents upper respiratory infection and lowers blood sugar levels.[38-40]

Laughter also reduces the perception of pain.[3,16,23,39,41] The exact mechanism of this effect remains unknown, although it is theorized that laughter stimulates the brain to release endorphins.[2,17-19] Endorphins are hormones that act as the body's natural pain killers. In addition, endorphins give people happy feelings and sometimes even feelings of euphoria, feelings that are produced when they laugh.

Relaxation Phase

People feel terrific after a good laugh. Following arousal and the release of hormones, the body responds automatically by relaxing muscular tensions.[30] In addition, blood pressure and heart rate drop below the pre-laughter rate. Laughter promotes breathing patterns that use the diaphragm, the opposite of the thoracic breathing that occurs under stress. Diaphragmatic breathing patterns produce respiratory relaxation.[1] The physical state of muscle relaxation cannot exist simultaneously with anxiety.[20,42,43]

PSYCHOLOGICAL EFFECTS OF LAUGHTER AND HUMOR

Humor and laughter can lead to beneficial psychological effects as well, especially emotional release. Humor helps people manage stress by enabling the release of nervous tensions. It offers an acceptable outlet for anxiety, fear, and anger. When people are anxious and fearful, they might shake and perspire to release pent-up emotions, characteristics of the flight component of the stress response. If, however, people can talk and laugh about anxiety and fear, they can obtain emotional relief. Similarly, when people are angry, their bodies seek to get rid of the emotional tension created by the anger. They feel hostile and resentful and may rant and rave, or they may lash out at someone or something. This is the fight component of the stress response, to attain release from anger. Or they can laugh and talk about the anger to release emotional tensions.[1,6,7,16]

Without the release of painful emotions, physical, emotional, and mental signs of stress develop. For example, people may feel nauseated (a physical sign), irritable (an emotional sign), and unable to concentrate (a mental sign). Excessive tension and a lack of therapeutic emotional release can bring on or aggravate many physical diseases, such as heart disease, diabetes, and ulcers. This reflects the wisdom in the popular phrase "You'll worry yourself sick." Most important to recognize is that communication becomes impaired, which may lead to misunderstandings and increase the risk for harmful events.

Laughter and humor, combined with meaningful verbal conversation, can produce the same beneficial relaxation, without the side effects of drugs, such as sedation and drowsiness. The advantage of humor and laughter with verbalization is that the patient maintains the ability to communicate, can think clearly, and is better able to collaborate in care and problem solving.

HOW PATIENTS USE HUMOR

The humorous messages sent from patients to nurses typically involve situations too painful to communicate directly. Strong negative emotions, such as fear, anger, and loss, may be defused through humor. Thus, humor is often used as indirect communication between the patient and nurse and, many times, it is used by patients to deliver very serious messages. So listen carefully, then think about and respond to the message behind the humor. If you fail to pick up on the meaning behind a humorous message, you risk increasing the emotional distance between yourself and the patient, and you will find yourself less effective in helping the patient deal with the situation and will increase the potential for a harmful event to occur. This section also covers gender differences in using humor.

Emotional Situations

There are many emotional situations that patients are forced to encounter in health-care settings. Sometimes, patients try to face (or avoid) such situations using humor. Patients often express their fears and concerns about body image through jokes. For example, suppose you are taking vital signs on a patient who had cardiac surgery 3 days ago and has been progressing very well. She is a tiny, thin lady who is 78 years old and is covered with dark bruises around her chest and leg incisions, around the sites used to obtain blood samples from both arms, and around the area where the central line had been inserted. The patient is sitting up in bed and, with smiling bright blue eyes, she looks at you and jokingly says, "Just look at me! It looks like someone beat me with a hammer."

You smile at her and say, "We sure do beat patients up around here, no doubt about it!" Then seriously you say, "I'll bet you're wondering if you are ever going to heal from all this. But you know, those black and blue marks are all normal, and they will all go away. Your incisions are also healing nicely, and your blood pressure and heart are doing fine."

Why did the patient make the joking remark? She was asking indirectly, "How am I doing? I look and feel a mess. Will I ever get better from all this?" This remark points to body image disturbance and a need for reassurance.

Embarrassing Situations

Embarrassing situations are numerous in health-care settings, including many that involve intimate procedures. Patients commonly joke about bedpans, bathrooms, and enemas to release nervous tension. Sometimes self-ridicule is used by the patient. For example, "How is a person with a big butt like mine supposed to fit on that bedpan?" Laughing with the patient would be appropriate. What if you had made that comment, "How is someone with a big butt like yours supposed to use this bedpan?" The patient almost certainly would have taken it as an insult. When a patient engages in self-ridicule, then you can laugh—gently—with the patient.

Patients may be embarrassed to talk about certain subjects and may initiate a topic through humor to determine whether it is acceptable to talk about. For example, suppose you are teaching a 55-year-old male patient with a colostomy how to irrigate and change the bag. In the middle of the irrigation, he laughs and says, "There goes my sex life! I guess I can work on my golf game." You smile at him and ask seriously, "Do you have some concerns about sex?" He responds, "My wife has such a weak stomach, she won't even look at this thing on me!"

You continue to let him express his feelings; then you say, "Maybe we can sit down with your wife and discuss this problem together." If you have little experience or knowledge in this area, then you can make a referral to other nurses on your unit or to another health-care provider. Nurses are not expected to be marriage counselors unless they have special certification, so it may be appropriate to assess the situation from the wife's perspective and then make a referral.

Unpleasant Situations

Unpleasant situations for patients are common in health-care settings. Patients often make jokes about their lack of control over what is being done to them and about the hospital routines. They pretend to be in a motel, and they joke about the food and the service they receive. You have seen many such jokes on the fronts of humorous get-well cards. These jokes are expressions of patients' feelings of powerlessness and lack of control. Listen to the message that the patient is really delivering. Joke back, and then become serious about the topic.

Some patients need to have blood drawn morning, noon, and night. They refer to the blood drawers as the "vampires." As you go to assess your patient, he says jokingly, "Those vampires keep coming to get me. They're sucking all my blood." You sense that he is angry and feels out of control, and you say, "The vampires do come in here a lot, but we need to know the results of all those tests. Do you have some questions about the blood tests?"

The patient says, "I just don't understand why they can't draw it once a day instead of so many times each day." Now you can explain the tests and what they indicate, and you can get him involved in what is being done. That should help decrease his feelings of anger and powerlessness.

Avoidance Tactic

Sometimes patients use humor to avoid facing problems. In this case, however, humor becomes maladaptive. Patients who constantly make jokes will not admit or express their true feelings. In this case, humor is used to escape from reality and to avoid confronting and dealing with fears. In other words, humor becomes a way of escaping from difficulties rather than making it easier to deal with difficulties by putting them in a new perspective. In this situation, you will probably need to confront the patient, help the patient take a serious look at the situation, and do some problem solving.

Sexually Oriented Humor

Men have a tendency to use sexually oriented humor in health-care situations more so than women. For instance, men may use sexually oriented jokes and teasing with female staff members. By doing so, they are asserting the masculinity that is threatened during hospitalization, especially if they perceive themselves to be dependent and powerless. They will make flirting comments and try to relate as a man to a woman rather than as a patient to a professional nurse.

Keep in mind that the basis for these comments is the threat to the male ego created by the situation. Do not think that you have done anything to encourage him. Instead of becoming embarrassed or defensive, respond with appropriate banter, and then assess the threat the patient is probably feeling.[13,17-19,44] Suppose you are giving the patient a back rub, and he says to you, "How about rubbing down a little lower." You could laugh and playfully tap him on the back and say, "I guess you are feeling well enough to be getting out of here. The sooner the better, I think!" Then say, seriously, "It's very difficult to be in the hospital when there are so many other things I'm sure you'd rather be doing." Now you have recognized the need behind the comment, the threat of dependency and feelings of powerlessness. If you have concerns about sexually oriented comments from male or female patients, it is appropriate to consult a nursing supervisor.

❖ HOW NURSES USE HUMOR

Humor in nursing is bound to the context of the situation. In all circumstances, jokes and funny stories must be fitting to the nursing situation and never insulting. It is important to know something about the patient, even to know the patient well, before you can judge whether the patient will appreciate the humor you see in a situation.

Usually, if a patient initiates humor by making a humorous remark, you can be almost certain that the patient will appreciate your similar response. Joking by nurses often involves playful, light-hearted teasing done with a cheerful attitude.[12,13,16] Nurses use humor to make contact with patients, maintain patient relationships, give patients hopes, educate patients, and maintain personal emotional stability.

Making Contact

As a nurse, you cannot be effective until you form a trusting relationship with the patient. Humor is one way of developing that relationship through sharing and expressing thoughts and feelings, including anxieties, fears, and anger. Demonstrating a sense of humor as you meet a patient can also serve to break the ice. When you share laughter with someone, you can quickly make supportive emotional contact.[1,5,43]

For example, consider the patient who comes in for a clinic visit, and you need to ask her to remove all her clothes and put on a flimsy paper gown. She is walking and talking and does not appear to be anxious, fearful, or in pain. Most people feel embarrassed and uncomfortable without clothes, however. So you comment, "Today, just for you, we have a stunning gown to wear during your examination! Isn't it lovely?"

You have demonstrated your sense of humor in an attempt to put the patient at ease and recognize verbally that you know most people are embarrassed by nakedness. You have shown your empathy in a witty manner. The patient responds with a smile and says, "I really hate these gowns, you know. And the whole thought of a physical worries me."

You have made contact, and the patient told you how she felt. Do you know what to say next? Remember to pick up on the emotion, using empathy. You become serious, and look her in the eyes and say, "Oh? What are you worried about?"

Maintaining Relationships

As you continue a relationship with a patient, humor helps put the person at ease and may increase cooperation with what you ask the person to do. When you need to give an injection, for example, you might say, "I have a soft and little needle for you because you're one of my favorite patients. I promise only a tiny pinch. Let's get this done. I'll be very quick about it." You are implying, "Relax, this isn't so terrible. You can trust me."

Or before sending a patient to surgery, you could jest, "Have a nice trip. We'll keep your bed warm for you, and we'll see you in a little bit." All patients going off to surgery are nervous about it. Humor keeps that anxiety in check. You give a patient confidence by these remarks.

Giving Patients Hope

Sometimes patients get depressed and may say to themselves, "This whole situation is hopeless. There's nothing I can do anymore that I like to do. I'll never get better." The inability to see options is characteristic of hopelessness and stress. Humor helps alter this narrow perspective and reframe a situation. It also helps to restore a sense of motivation.

A nurse came to take the pulse of an elderly patient who had just had major surgery. He loved to play bocce ball at the senior citizen club. The patient told the nurse, "I won't be able to play anymore." The nurse tried to reassure him verbally without success. But after taking his pulse, the nurse said, "I can tell you're a bocce ball player from your heartbeat." He looked surprised and then smiled. "You really think I'll be able to play again?"

In this situation, the patient's depression was not so severe that his affect was frozen. He was able to respond to the warmth and caring the nurse's humor conveyed. The idea is that if a patient can take a detached view of a situation, the patient can think more objectively and can begin to solve problems.

Patient Education

Humor stimulates people physically and mentally, and its use may make patients more receptive to information and increase their willingness to explore and analyze new ideas.[45] Humor can be used to strengthen major points or basic ideas that must be conveyed to the patient during teaching. Humorous information can often be remembered longer and more easily than information presented in a formal manner. Humorous analogies, anecdotes, and parables can help teach family planning and health concepts.[46]

For example, you might write humorous expressions related to a class topic on name tags, and then have the patients choose a name tag at the beginning of class. The patients can introduce themselves and explain why they chose their particular humorous expression.[47] These name tags can be used as ice breakers to help establish a warm and congenial environment, to set the tone for the class, and to put the patients at ease.

Emotional Stability

You can also use humor with other nurses to distance yourself from pain and suffering. In fact, nurses commonly use a macabre form of humor that people outside of nursing may not find funny. Here is an example. The evening intensive care unit (ICU) nurses were sitting at the conference table and had just finished hearing the day shift's patient report. One of the night nurses had called in sick, and there was no one to replace her. It was going to be a long evening without enough staff and very busy. Eight of 11 patients in the medical ICU were on ventilators, unconscious, and in critical condition. One remarked to the others, "We're working in a vegetable garden tonight." The others laughed, and another nurse said, "Well, everyone grab your shovels and buckets, and let's get to work. We're good. We'll get through it." Everyone laughed again.

The joking relieved the frustration by detaching them from the situation. It was a good thing that no family members were around to hear this grim humor. Freud described this as gallows humor, where individuals laugh at death and tragedy to help cope with a morbid situation.[43,48-50]

CHAPTER SUMMARY

Humor and laughter are cost-effective and time-effective patient-safe communication strategies that can be used for health promotion. Nurses are finding ways to use humor and laughter as a means to communicate effectively with patients and prevent patient harm.

Like other patient-safe strategies, nures need to practice using humor if it is to become integrated into communications within nurse-patient relationships. You must expand your sense of humor by developing an attitude that allows you to see the absurdities in situations, others, and especially in yourself.

Still, what is considered funny and amusing to one person may be insulting, tasteless, embarrassing, or emotionally painful to another. It is important never to be insulting with humor and to assess each patient carefully for physical and emotional discomforts before using humor to promote nurse-patient relationships.

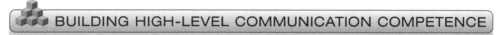 BUILDING HIGH-LEVEL COMMUNICATION COMPETENCE

For additional exercises, visit DavisPlus at http://davisplus.fadavis.com

Critical Thinking: Analyze the following "jokes" to determine what the patient is really trying to tell you. What would be an appropriate response to each one?

As you clear his uneaten dinner, a 50-year-old male patient says with a smile, "That was the most delicious food in the world. My compliments to the chef."

A 30-year-old male patient recovering from an appendectomy says, "Hey, honey, how about some hug therapy?"

An 88-year-old woman rocks in her chair and chants, "Oh dear, oh dear, if I were dead, I wouldn't be here." She is smiling, alert, and oriented.

A surgeon removed the belly button of an 84-year-old woman as he repaired her umbilical hernia. When he makes rounds the next day, she quips to him, "You're a shoemaker! Now, how is my husband supposed to recognize me when I get to heaven?"

A 50-year-old woman who just had a mastectomy states, "All those things ever did was get in the way!"

A 62-year-old woman tells the neurosurgeon after a craniotomy, "You're a good surgeon but a lousy barber!"

References

1. Dugan, D.O. Laughter and Tears: Best Medicine for Stress. Nursing Forum 24:18, 1989.
2. Hoesl, N.L. Laughter: The Drug of Choice: Definitive Doses of the Best Medicine, 2nd ed. Cincinnati, Ohio, LaughterDoc Publications: 2007.
3. Cousins, N. The Anatomy of an Illness, N.Y., Norton: 1979.
4. Cousins, N. The Anatomy of an Illness as Perceived by the Patient: Reflections on Healing and Regeneration, N.Y., Norton: 2005.
5. Fosbinder, D. Patient Perceptions of Nursing Care: An Emerging Theory of Interpersonal Competence. Journal of Advanced Nursing 20:1085, 1994.
6. McGhee, P. Rx: Laughter. RN 98:50, 1998.
7. McGhee, P. Health, Healing, and the Amuse System. Dubuque, Iowa, Kendall/Hunt: 1996.
8. Fonnesbeck, B.G. Are You Kidding? Nursing98 28:64, 1998.

9. Astedt-Kurki, P., Isola, A. Humour Between Nurse and Patient and Among Staff: Analysis of Nurses' Diaries. Journal of Advanced Nursing 35:452-458, 2001.
10. Astedt-Kurki, P.I.A., Tammertie, T., Kervinen, U. Importance of Humour to Client-Nurse Relationships and Clients' Well-Being. International Journal of Nursing Practice 7:119-125, 2001.
11. Dean, R.A., Gregory D. More Than Trivial: Strategies for Using Humor in Palliative Care. Cancer Nursing 28:292-300, 2005.
12. Wanzer, M., Booth-Butterfield, M., Booth-Butterfield, S. If We Didn't Use Humor, We'd Cry: Humourous Coping Communication in Health Care Settings. Journal of Health Communication 10:105-125, 2005.
13. Finch, L.P. Patients' Communication With Nurses: Relational Communication and Preferred Nurse Behaviors. International Journal for Human Caring 10:14-22, 2006.
14. McCreaddie, M., Wiggins, S. The Purpose and Function of Humour in Health, Health Care and Nursing: A Narrative Review. Journal of Advanced Nursing, 61:584-595, 2007.
15. Association for Applied and Therapeutic Humor. Located at: http://www.aath.org/ Accessed December, 2008.
16. MacDonald, P. Laughter—The Best Medicine? Practice Nurse 36:38-39, 2008.
17. Robinson, V: Humor and Health. In McGhee, P.E., Goldstein, J.H. (eds.). Handbook of Humor Research, vol. 2. N.Y., Springer-Verlag, 1983, p 109.
18. Robinson, V.M. Humor and the Health Professions, 2nd ed. Thorofare, N.J. Slack Inc., 1991.
19. Robinson, V. Humor in Nursing. In Carlson, C., Blackwell, B. (eds.). Behavioral Concepts and Nursing Intervention, 2nd ed. Philadelphia, J.B. Lippincott: 1978.
20. Chinery, W. Alleviating Stress With Humor: A Literature Review. Journal of Perioperative Practice 17:172-182, 2007.
21. Westburg, N.G. Hope, Laughter and Humor in Residents and Staff at an Assisted Living Facility. Journal of Mental Health Nursing 25:16-32, 2003.
22. Schmitt, N. Patients' Perception of Laughter in a Rehabilitation Hospital. Rehabilitation Nursing 1:143, 1990.
23. Astedt-Kurki, P. Humour in Nursing Care. Journal of Advanced Nursing 20:183,1994.
24. Astedt-Kurki, P., Haggman-Laitila, A. Good Nursing Practice as Perceived by Clients: A Starting Point to the Development of Professional Nursing. Journal of Advanced Nursing 17:1195, 1992.
25. Calman, L. Patients' Views of Nurses' Competence. Nurse Education Today 26:719-725, 2006.
26. Fenwick, C.R. Love and Laughter: A Healing Journey. Muenster, SK, Canada, St. Peter's Press: 2004.
27. Morreall, J. Taking Laughter Seriously. Albany, N.Y., State University of New York Press: 1983.
28. Morreall, J. Humor Works. Amherst, Mass., HRD Press: 1997.
29. Pasquali, E.A. Learning to Laugh: Humor as Therapy. Journal of Psychosocial Nursing 28:31,1990.
30. Martin, R.A. The Psychology of Humor: An Integrative Approach. London, Elsevier: 2006.
31. Ruxton, J.P. Humor Intervention Deserves Our Attention. Holistic Nursing Practice 2:54,1988.
32. Berk, L.S., Tan, S.A. Immune System Changes During Humor Associated With Laughter. Clinical Research 39:124A, 1991.
33. Berk, L.S., Tan, S.A., Fry, W. Eustress of Humor-Associated Laughter Modulates Specific Immune System Components. Annals of Behavioral Medicine 15(Suppl):S111, 1993.
34. Berk, L.S., Tan, S.A. A Positive Emotion, the Eustress of Mirthful Laughter Modulates the Immune System Lymphokine Interferon-Gamma. Psychoneuroimmunology Research Society Annual Meetings, April (Abstract Supplement) 5:A1, 1995.
35. Kimata, H. Differential Effects of Laughter on Allergen-Specific Immunoglobulin and Neurotrophin Levels in Tears. Perceptual and Motor Skills 98:901-908, 2004.
36. Kimata, H. Effects of Humor on Allergen-Induced Wheal Reactions. Journal of the American Medical Association 286:737, 2001.
37. Mazer, E. Ten Sure-Fire Stress Releasers. Prevention 34:104,1989.
38. Diamond, J. Your Body Doesn't Lie. N.Y.,Warner: 1979.
39. Siegel, B. Love, Medicine, and Miracles. N.Y., Harper Perennial: 1990.
40. Hayashi, K., Hayashi, T., Iwangaga, S., et al. Laughter Lowered the Increase in Postprandial Blood Glucose. Diabetes Care 26:1651-1652, 2003.
41. Nevo, O., Keinan, G., Teshimousky-Ardit, M. Humor and Pain Tolerance. International Journal of Humor Research 6:71, 1993.
42. Flavier, J.M. The Lessons of Laughter. World Health Forum 11:412, 1990.
43. Samra, C. A Time to Laugh. Journal of Christian Nursing 3:17, 1985.
44. Lippert, L., Hunt S. An Ethnographic Study of the Role of Humor in Health Care Transactions. Lewiston, N.Y., Edwin Mellen Press: 2005.
45. Freud, S. Jokes and Their Relationship to the Unconscious. In Strachey, J. (ed.). The Complete Psychological Works of Sigmund Freud, vol 8. London, Hogarth Press: 1961.

46. Bastable, S.B. Nurse as Educator: Principles of Teaching and Learning for Nursing Practice, 3rd ed. Sudbury, Mass., Jones & Bartlett: 2008.
47. White, L.A., Lewis, D.J. Humor: A Teaching Strategy to Promote Learning. Journal of Nursing Staff Development 3:60,1990.
48. Williams, H. Humour and Healing: Therapeutic Effects in Geriatrics. Gerontion 1:14,1986.
49. Freud, S. Humor. International Journal of Psychoanalysis 9:1, 1928.
50. Parfitt, J.M. Humorous Preoperative Teaching. Association of Perioperative Registered Nurses Journal 52:114, 1990.

Nurse-Patient Relationships During Grief, Mourning, and Loss

Learning Outcomes

Upon completion of this chapter, you will be able to:

1. Explain the relationship among grief, mourning, loss, and tears.
2. Identify the losses that occur at each stage of growth and development.
3. Describe how tears promote emotional healing.
4. Describe the physiological processes that occur with the release of tears.
5. List reasons why people cry.
6. Describe gender and cultural differences in crying.
7. Identify appropriate patient-safe strategies and inappropriate nursing responses during grief, mourning, loss, and tears.

Key Words

Grief
Anticipatory grieving
Mourning

Sadness
Loss
Depression

The purpose of this chapter is to explore patient responses during times of grief, mourning, and loss and appropriate patient-safe strategies as responses to be used within the nurse-patient relationship. A primary focus of this chapter is applying patient-safe communication strategies when a patient or family member cries and during grief, mourning, and loss. These strategies include establishing trust and rapport, using perception checking, and using empathy and other facilitative listening responses. Review the Transformational Model of Communication in Chapter 2, and locate grief, mourning, and loss in the risk factor ring, along with trust and rapport, perception checking, empathy, and facilitative listening responses in the patient-safe strategies ring. *For an interactive version of this activity, see DavisPlus at http://davisplus.fadavis.com*

The purpose of the exercise is to introduce you to one of the main human responses during grief, mourning, and loss: crying. Many student nurses are uncomfortable when a patient or family member cries, until they learn that crying and tears are nature's way of allowing a person to release tension from the body and to communicate a need to be comforted.[1] This chapter describes the loss that occurs during each phase of growth and development throughout the life span, the purposes of crying and tears, and patient-safe strategies to promote positive transformational outcomes. In addition, this chapter discusses what *not* to say when patients and family members cry and concludes with a section on what to do as a nurse when you become close to patients and experience grief along with them.

GRIEF

Grief involves a process that all people experience, usually after the death of a loved one or another significant loss. Grief is an intense and painful emotional state. Grief work involves the process of working through the emotional reaction to loss and reorganizing lifestyles to accommodate the loss. The emotional reaction may last for an extended period. After the loss of a pet, a person may experience 20 hours of crying. The loss of a spouse, parent, child, or close friend may result in 200 or 300 hours of crying. Tears are common even years after the loss of someone who has been very close.[2,3] Anticipatory grief occurs before an actual loss, usually during a long terminal illness.

Communication Safety Alert

Tears are beneficial. Tears release the sadness, anger, hate, and guilt commonly present with anticipatory grief. In early grief, talking through tears about the final days with the deceased and reviewing good and bad memories can be therapeutic.

A major loss means that the person must modify his or her belief system to fit a new reality. The new reality is that the person must restructure his or her life without the loved one who died. In a grief reaction to significant loss, a person might say, "I just don't know what to believe in anymore."

Loss requires a person to say good-bye to someone who has been very important to them. It does not mean to forget or diminish the value of the loved one who died. It means closing the door on what was lost and opening a new door to a new life without the loved one. The grieving person must learn to cope with the loss. Triumph over the loss means the person still sees a purpose in living and again becomes actively involved in meaningful activities.[1,4,5]

Old relationships are modified, and new ones are formed. As time passes, sadness turns into loneliness and eventually into hopefulness. The focus is less on the loss and more on the changes needed to adjust. Successful resolution of the loss gives the survivor a greater understanding of life with greater compassion for suffering and a higher sensitivity to the needs of others.

Grief Work

A grieving person should be allowed to choose whether he or she wants to be around others and participate in activities. The person may need a period of denial and withdrawal. Too long a period, however, may lead to hyperactivity, hostility, depression, changes in relationships with others, and overall decreased ability to function. A grief counselor or support group may be needed to help the patient grieve the loss. A patient who has suffered a loss should be encouraged to grieve and continue to have the emotional support of health-care professionals, family, and friends until the grieving is finished.[1,4-6]

Communication Safety Alert

Grieving for the death of a loved one may extend over a year and up to 3 years. Throughout grieving, certain people, objects, and occasions evoke memories of the deceased, bringing on feelings of sadness and depression, often with resultant tears to relieve the feelings.[1,4-6]

Chronic Stress and Depression Associated With Grief and Loss

Chronic stress occurs with unresolved grief and loss, and sadness turns into depression—emotional depression and physiological depression of the immune system. Thus, affected people are more susceptible to colds and flu, and they can have symptoms of emotional depression and stress, such as fatigue, headaches, and backaches.[1] Over time, chronic stress leads to diseases such as hypertension, gastric reflux, and indigestion. Unexpressed grief over loss negatively affects behavior and emotional well-being when people become unable to function in their personal lives or their jobs.

LOSSES EXPERIENCED THROUGHOUT STAGES OF LIFE

All people experience loss as they go through each stage of their lives. Every loss involves emotional tensions and sadness with which individuals must learn to cope in order to maintain emotional and physical health. If people can learn to recognize and grieve appropriately for small losses, they will be prepared better to deal with the big losses that occur.[4,5] Therefore, the next section covers the losses that occur in each stage of growth and development, beginning with childhood at the stage when the child becomes cognitively aware of missing someone or something.

Childhood

During early childhood, any separation from the parents is a loss. The child does not know that the parents will return but eventually gains an understanding that parents will return and that the child can love and trust people other than parents. As the child grows, he or she becomes increasingly independent. Entering preschool and kindergarten is exciting and frightening because the child loses the security of home, although new experiences, friends, and teachers are gained.

Throughout school, the child is promoted from grade to grade, losing familiar teachers and gaining new ones. Friendships break up because interests change, classmates move, or the child may move. Developmental tasks include becoming autonomous from parents, taking the initiative to try new things, and becoming industrious and winning recognition for achievements at school and in extracurricular activities. Children learn to be industious workers at school and home, developing many self-care skills and gradually becoming more self-sufficient.[6-9]

Adolescence

Promotions to middle school and high school mean giving up many childhood things. Adolescent life events include establishing relationships with members of the opposite sex, graduating, and getting a job. When a relationship ends, teens may feel intense loss, even if the relationship was not sexual and they both agreed to end it. Graduation is a happy event, but it results in the breaking up of many relationships and, in many cases, leaving home. A job is a significant gain of a new role and an income. If a job is terminated, however, the role and income are lost. The relatively carefree life of childhood and adolescence ends as the adolescent takes on adult responsibilities. The major developmental task of adolescence is to develop a sense of identity and to decide on a career.[6-9]

Young Adulthood

The young adult struggles for financial independence, starts a career, forms close sexual relationships, starts a family, and sets up a home. Each event has the potential for satisfaction and happiness but also has the potential for loss. These losses can come from being fired; from being divorced; from sustaining property damage through fire, theft, flood, or other disaster; from moving and the consequent loss of friends and their support; and from the death of friends or family members. The major developmental task of young adulthood is to develop intimacy in relationships, develop a career, and start a family.[6-9]

Middle Age

During the middle adult years, many people find enjoyment in the fruits of their labors but the gains and losses of life continue. Sometimes a promotion means increased salary and prestige but a loss of free time. Expenses peak as children reach college age. A real sense of loss occurs as children leave home to attend school, marry, or get their own apartments. Parents welcome the growing independence of their children, but they experience a loss that the children no longer need them in the same ways. The parent-child relationship changes to an adult-adult relationship. As the last child leaves home, many parents—especially mothers—experience a well-known depressive event called the "empty nest syndrome." Although they are joyful at a child's independence, parents miss having the child around as much, and the daily relationship with the child must change. Also, the role of a parent with children to raise is over.

Sometimes in middle adulthood, people realize that they may not be able to achieve all the goals they aspired to in their youth. They experience a sense of loss. At some point, a person in middle age faces the realization of lost youth. There are changes in body proportions, wrinkles, vision changes, gray hair, sometimes baldness, and the loss of physical stamina. Women must adapt to menopause and the loss of fertility. Although a man's sexual function can continue into his 80s, temporary dysfunction may become more evident at middle age and may be traumatic.

Many middle-aged adults adapt to and accept the effects of time. Others experience a midlife crisis and set out to prove that they are still young. Divorces occur as one partner seeks out younger companions. Middle age is especially difficult for people who emphasize youth and sex appeal as a way of life. A major task of middle adults is generativity, which involves guiding the next generation through home, work, and community activities.[6-9]

Late Adulthood

In late adulthood, losses far outnumber gains. There is continued physical decline in all organ systems, the most noticeable being visual and hearing losses, difficulties with mobility, and loss of memory. Friends and family members are lost through moving and death. Retirement can be viewed as a significant loss of productive activity, loss of income, and loss of relationships.

When a person is deemed no longer able to drive or no longer able to live alone, there is a loss of independence, which most elderly people fear keenly. Moving to a retirement home or nursing home involves the loss of one's home and all that was familiar in that environment. After major losses, many people experience a significant decline in health.

In preparation for death, even though life has been very productive and full, elderly people fear losing their minds, losing control of their lives, becoming a burden, and having more pain than they can bear. The primary task of the older adult is to develop a sense of ego integrity in which the person can look back on life with a sense of satisfaction and acceptance of impending death.[6-9]

Learning how to deal with loss is one of life's most difficult and most important lessons. At each stage of growth and development, people must learn to recognize their feelings and then work through the emotions as they react to the losses.

Communication Safety Alert

Depending on the loss and its meaning to the individual, a person may also experience a loss of security, self-esteem, a belief system, or faith.

The Impact of Illness on Growth and Development

Now imagine what happens when someone at any stage of life becomes seriously ill (or dies). The patient and family have been picked up out of the typical daily struggles and thrown into a crisis. The meaning of and response to the crisis vary with the growth and development of the person and family before the crisis. The usual growth and development tasks are interrupted. Illness results in altered roles and relationships. The resulting nursing care will be focused on how to help patients and families adjust to altered roles and relationships and on how to help patients and families grieve their losses. Nurses must recognize that it takes time to grieve and that everyone has the right to grieve for the losses, big and small.

During an illness, a person may grieve for the loss of body image, such as with a mastectomy. Nursing students must understand the typical struggles of psychological growth and development and assess the growth and development of patients prior to the present health situation. Once you understand what was going on in their lives, you recognize that patients may have experienced significant losses that affect the current situation. Thus, you develop patient and family background data to form the basis for showing empathy and understanding the meaning of sickness or death to patients and family members in their current situation.

One of the most typical patient responses to grief, mourning, and loss is crying. Before describing patient-safe strategies used to promote postive transformational outcomes, you must understand the nature and meaning of crying and tears. People shed tears for many specific reasons, but there is usually some form of loss involved.

WHY PEOPLE CRY

People cry when they grieve and mourn the loss of a loved one. But there are many other times people cry. Many people cry at weddings, graduations, or when moving to a newer and bigger home, even though these are happy events. The sadness is caused by the losses that will result from the happy event. The father of the bride "gives his little girl away," and his relationship with his daughter under his care and protection is over. She is starting a new family and new chapter of life in marriage. At the same time, the father and daughter and other family members may be remembering a loved one who they wish could have lived to see the event, thus resulting in sadness.

Tears are also shed due to feelings of frustration and anger. A person may be angry about a situation he cannot seem to resolve, or she is trying very hard to do something but without success. Frustrations and anger occur in everday situations. Perhaps the person is feeling embarrassed and humiliated. In these situations, the person feels a sense of loss because the person has not lived up to self-expectations. Crying may help to relieve the tension.

Sometimes people cry because they are frightened. They do not know if an outcome will be good or if they will be able to cope with a situation. For example, a patient may be afraid of the outcomes of diangostic testing. A patient who earlier had a computerized tomographic scan may cry and say, "I'm afraid the tests will show I have cancer." The person fears the changes that may occur in lifestyle if the diagnosis of cancer is confirmed. The person also fears death.

People also cry when they are in pain, either because they hurt or because the pain frightens them. Pain means that something is wrong, and something wrong means that people can no longer do what they would rather be doing. Thus, in a sense, pain is also a loss, the loss of ability to perform activites. People are afraid of pain, especially if they do not know how to manage it, what is causing it, or how much damage has been done to their body.

Tears can be used as weapons, however. During conflict, tears can be manipulative and have a controlling intent. As a result of manipulation, all involved can feel increased frustration, tension, and alienation.[2,3] For example, suppose you do not want to do something for someone, and as a result, the other person begins to cry. Then you feel guilty, selfish, and sorry for the other person. You agree to do what the person wants, but you feel resentful because you feel manipulated and controlled. You have assumed the role of placator. You need to use assertive and active listening patient-safe communication strategies to manage a situation when the intent of a person's tears is to manipulate and control.

In most circumstances, people shed tears to release tensions that are associated with loss. Tensions associated with loss lead to such physiological symptoms as tightness in the chest, choking, shortness of breath, sighing, empty feelings in the stomach, and feelings of weakness.[1,10] These feelings are very distressing. Tears must flow in order to release such tensions and to resolve the physiological ramifications.

A "Good" Cry

Weeping helps a person feel better because tears can reduce perceived emotional pain levels and can actually create pleasant sensations. Tears are therapeutic because they are a cathartic coping mechanism that helps resolve feelings of loss, grief, fear, frustration, and anger. There are chemicals in tears that help to reduce stress.[1,11,12] If the tears are shut off and the emotional pain is ignored, the tensions are not released, and the waste chemicals excreted in tears remain trapped in the body. It is also healthy to release tensions through tears in close relationships. Tears can break down barriers and build stronger bonds in relationships.[11,12]

By releasing stress-related tensions and hormones, crying produces a relaxation response. Initially, tears stimulate the sympathetic nervous system, causing the release of catecholamines that increase blood pressure and heart rate. This arousal is followed by a parasympathetic response that generates a state of systemic relaxation. Sobbing leads to respiratory relaxation by producing diaphragmatic breathing patterns instead of the thoracic tension-producing breathing pattern associated with the fight-or-flight response. We feel "pleasantly drained" after a good long cry.[2,3]

GENDER DIFFERENCES IN SHEDDING TEARS

Gender differences in communication are the focus of Chapter 5. This section further expands on the specific concept of gender and crying. Women commonly vent their tensions, anger, and frustrations by crying. Men commonly vent by yelling and shouting.[1,11,12]

It is interesting to note that women in all societies cry more than men, possibly because of hormonal differences in the genders. Women secrete 30 times more of the hormone prolactin than men. Prolactin is involved chemically with secretions of milk and tears. It is believed that women cry more than men do, in part, because of their increased prolactin levels.[2,3]

There is also cultural pressure for men not to cry; crying is considered not "manly." This is clearly delineated in the expression "You're a big boy. Big boys don't cry." In contrast, girls are permitted to cry and express themselves. Thus, male and female children have been culturally conditioned to respond differently. Men experience just as much emotional turmoil as women; however, men are taught not to cry as readily.

Men generally tend not to open up as much as women. They tend to hold their feelings inside and reveal less personal information when they are emotionally overwhelmed and will tend to stifle their tears. Men are, however, beginning to recognize the importance of crying in releasing pent-up emotions and dealing with stress. Men and boys are being encouraged to show their emotions and not to be afraid to let out tears of true emotion.[11,12] Men are realizing that crying shows sensitivity and is acceptable.

PATIENT-SAFE STRATEGIES IN RESPONSE TO CRYING

You can encourage patients and families to express themselves to help ease feelings of sadness, loss, and grief. Your role as a compassionate health-care professional is to help patients recognize that crying is not a sign of weakness or inadequacy but rather is a communication mechanism that enables the patient to mourn life losses actively. Patients value the supportive presence of the nurse and feelings of outside acceptance related to the flow of tears.

Communication Safety Alert

Use of empathy and facilitative listening are the main patient-safe communication strategies as described in earlier chapters. Health-care providers need to allow the expression of tears to relieve tension, and then listen to the patients' feelings and concerns.

For example, during rounds you find an elderly woman patient sitting in bed with tears in her eyes and on her cheeks. You have no idea what could be the matter. Without any other information to go on, you estimate at this point that she is mildly upset. The basic empathic approach is always to deal with the emotion first. Let the emotion be recognized. So you say, "I can see that you're upset," and offer her a tissue. Next, you sit down so you are on the same level with the patient. Make eye contact, and prepare to use active listening skills. Also use touch, such as a hug or a hand on the patient's hand or arm as you say, "What's going on?" or "What are these tears about?" Follow that with a smile and "I'm a good listener."

As the patient speaks, nod and use facilitators, such as restatement and clarification, to get a clear picture of the patient's view of her situation. Resist all temptation to interrupt, give advice, change the subject, or give a pep talk. Listen as she tells you as she continues to shed tears that she has a son who does not have time to come and see her as often as she would like. She explains that he is working and has his own family and that she misses him and his family. Her husband died a year ago as well, and she misses him, too. She adds, "I'm just sitting here feeling blue."

To respond with empathy, say something like, "I can see you miss them, and you're probably feeling a bit lonely." Then encourage her to talk about her son or her husband. For example, you could say, "When was the last time you saw your son or his family?" or "How long were you married?" You are showing your interest in her situation by asking these questions.

Although you can do nothing to change the patient's situation, you have helped her to feel better by allowing her to release emotions through tears and words. The patient recognizes that you care about her enough to take a few minutes to listen to her situation and empathize with her.

What about a person who is angry and weeps at the same time? Consider, for example, a 30-year-old woman who has been married for 5 years. She was in the gynecology clinic when she was told she had gonorrhea by the physician. The nurse was going to teach her about the disease, its transmission, its prevention, and the importance of obtaining information about her sexual partners. Just as the nurse began, the patient became angry and shouted, "How could he do this to me?" She was crying and cursing at the same time, as she paced back and forth. The nurse remained calm, without judging or arguing. The nurse showed acceptance of the crying and cursing, as she waited for the patient to regain control. Explosive emotions involve underlying feelings of helplessness and hurt.[1] The nurse's presence and silence were ways of showing acceptance while the patient was releasing emotional tension by blowing off steam. Silence also helps a patient collect her thoughts.

Then the patient sat down and began to sob. The nurse sat next to her and took her hand. "I know you're hurting," she said, recognizing verbally the pain the woman was feeling over her husband's betrayal. The patient was able to talk more calmly but was still crying, "I'm sorry I've behaved so badly. I just don't know what I'm supposed to do now." The nurse says, "I'm here for you, and we can figure out together what you can do now."

When someone is extremely upset and in great emotional pain, the emotions need to be expressed. Listen to the person's story with empathy. The nurse needs to be open and accepting so that the patient can release emotional tension and begin to think about the problem and what to do next.

Patient-Safe Communication Strategies to Help Families Grieve

Encouraging family members to talk to and touch a dying patient will help them to grieve their loss. It is very therapeutic for family members to share in the dying process, for both the patient and the family. Many dying patients say that their greatest fear is dying alone. They want family with them. For survivors, being with the patient in the final moments is therapeutic as well and facilitates the grief process. A common misbelief is that witnessing a death or viewing a body immediately after death is too traumatic. In actuality, this misbelief inhibits the grief process.

Hospitals can be very intimidating, and the family may want to stay out of the way. But in doing so, family members may miss the final opportunity to be with the dying person. Encourage close family members to stay with the patient and to talk and touch as much as possible throughout the dying process, even if the patient is comatose. In hospital settings, let the family provide as much care for the patient as they would like, such as bathing or shaving the patient. As an alternative, a terminally ill person may join a hospice program that provides palliative care throughout the dying process. The patient may be able to die at home if he or she chooses.

The best patient-safe communication strategy nurses can offer as health-care providers is acceptance. Use facilitative listening responses, and encourage patients to express their feelings. Encourage patients to work though an impending loss at their own speed. Check in on the patient and family, and let them know you are available. Offer food and drink to the family. Do all you can to provide comfort measures, and allow the patient as many choices as possible. As appropriate, offer to call the hospital chaplain or a pastor, priest, rabbi, or other spiritual leader of the patient's choice. Social workers can also help families deal with grief and will know which community resources are appropriate for the family.

WHAT NOT TO SAY WHEN A PATIENT CRIES

Many nurses feel uncomfortable when a patient cries; they feel bad about a patient's unpleasant situation and become upset and anxious. To reduce their own feelings of discomfort, these nurses may want to quiet the patient quickly. This minimizes the patient's cause for crying or expresses disapproval of the crying. Comments include, "There's no need to cry. You're doing fine." or "Let's stop crying now." By quieting the patient, the nurse spares herself the need to address her own emotional turmoil as well as that of the patient. Other responses intended to quiet a patient and bury emotions include such comments as, "Get hold of yourself" (advice), "Think positive" (more advice), "Think of your family" (guilt), "I promise that everything will be fine" (false reassurance), or "You shouldn't feel that way" (judgmental).

With respect to bereavement after the death of a loved one, people who prefer to avoid the emotions that result in crying may also choose certain expressions to convey condolences after the death of a loved one. These expressions deny the importance of the grief or imply that the person has no right to grieve the loss. These comments include, "You must be strong," which implies that only weak people show grief; "You must be a man about this," which implies that men and boys should not cry or grieve; and "It is time to get on with your life," which implies that grieving should consume a certain amount of time, after which the person no longer has a right to grieve.

Communication Safety Alert

If you can hear yourself making any of the above statements, then you do not understand—and are not trying to understand—the feelings of people who are crying. Your best course of action is to erase these comments permanently from your list of appropriate things to say when someone is crying or at any other time.

These remarks might help you feel better, but they are not patient-safe communication strategies of empathy and facilitative listening; they block expression of emotions; and the patient will not want to talk with you. You will silence the patient, and trust and rapport will be gone. In addition, as previously discussed, you should never offer false hope or make promises you cannot keep.

Sometimes, if, in a health-care provider's opinion, patients become too upset, crying and tears may be treated with medications. In some cases, medications may be useful if they help people become more ready to discuss problems. Overmedication does not allow, however, for the release of painful emotions and the examination of underlying emotional pain. Drugs may provide an easy way to quiet a person and perhaps help the person to sleep, but loss and grief remain unresolved. To help a patient resolve grief, a patient needs to be able to express feelings.

NURSES CRY, TOO

As a nurse, you may identify with situations that do not involve you personally. You will become emotionally involved, and you will cry. When caring for patients and families, you will become close to them and experience grief along with them.[13] You will cry—and should cry—to release the tensions associated with that grief.

Sometimes you will cry with patients and families; sometimes you will cry in private. It is important to recognize that when you cry, you are relieving your own emotional pain. Crying together with a patient or a family member can create a valuable and supportive bond. But you should avoid crying with a patient or family member unless that other person cries first. So what do you do when you feel like crying but need to remain in professional control? Get behind closed doors to a safe and private place to let out your emotions. Talk about your feelings with a trusted colleague, who has undoubtedly had similar feelings and can help you sort through yours.

Communication Safety Alert

Before you can help others undergoing grief and loss, it is important to recognize and acknowledge your own vulnerability to grief and loss.

You must acknowledge that you can never be in total control of your life and that some events are beyond your control. Once you make this acknowledgment, it is easier to deal with the fear, guilt, and anger caused by a loss over which you have no control. You must also acknowledge your own mortality and that life as you know it can end at any moment. We all recognize that not everyone lives to the average age of death, which is near 80 years. The reflection exercises at the end of the chapter are especially designed to help you as a health-care provider recognize your own vulnerability to grief and loss.

CHAPTER SUMMARY

This chapter describes grief, mourning, and loss that occur not only over the death of loved ones but also during each stage of growth and development throughout life. Tears are a natural and effective way to release the tension that accompanies sadness, grief, anger, and fear. A sense of loss is the overriding feeling that leads to crying and tears.

Nursing a patient who feels a loss involves helping the person to feel "bad." It means helping the patient experience painful emotions so that the person can experience the benefits of releasing tensions through tears. It also means listening supportively to the patient and family as they verbalize emotional pain. Patient-safe communication with a crying patient means that you avoid expressing disapproval or minimizing the cause for crying.

BUILDING HIGH-LEVEL COMMUNICATION COMPETENCE

For additional exercises, see DavisPlus at http://davisplus.fadavis.com

1. **Reflective Practice.** Write a one-page summary of a significant loss you experienced. You may describe any loss, such as the loss of body image, loss of a loved one, or loss of a job. What were your feelings during the experience? What were your behaviors during the experience? How did you resolve your feelings of loss?

2. **Critical Thinking.** Break the class into small groups to discuss and summarize the feelings, behaviors, and ways of resolving feelings of loss identified in the first exercise. Have a designated leader tell the class the summary findings from each group.

3. **Reflection.** Use the following exercise to think about your own mortality. Suppose you are in a car accident and die tomorrow. List the relationships that would be lost. What should be done with your body? Would you want a funeral or memorial service? What would you want done with your property? List the uncompleted tasks you would leave behind. List activities that you should not put off any longer.

References

1. Wolfelt, A.D. Companioning the Bereaved: A Soulful Guide for Caregivers. Fort Collins, Colo., Companion Press: 2006.
2. Dugan, D. Laughter and Tears: Best Medicine for Stress. Nursing Forum 24:18, 1989.
3. Lütz, T. Crying : The Natural and Cultural History of Tears. N.Y., Norton: 2001.
4. Kübler-Ross, E. To Live Until We Say Goodbye. Englewood Cliffs, N.J., Prentice-Hall: 1978.
5. Kübler-Ross, E., Kessler, D. On Grief and Grieving: Finding the Meaning of Grief Through the Five Stages. Riverside, N.J., Simon and Schuster: 2005.
6. Milliken, M.E. Understanding Human Behavior, 7th ed. Albany, N.Y., Delmar: 2004.
7. Erikson, E.H. Childhood and Society, 2nd ed. N.Y., Norton: 1963 (reissued 1993).
8. Erikson, E.H. The Life Cycle Completed. N.Y., Norton: 1998.
9. Harder, A.F. The Developmental Stages of Erik Erikson. Located at http://www.learningplaceonline.com/stages/organize/Erikson.htm Accessed January, 2009.
10. Schulz, R. The Psychology of Death, Dying, and Bereavement. Reading, Mass., Addison-Wesley: 1978.
11. Glass, L. He Says, She Says: Closing the Communication Gap Between the Sexes. N.Y., Berkley: 1993.
12. Glass, L. I Know What You're Thinking: Using the Four Codes of Reading People to Improve Your Life. Hoboken, N.J., John Wiley & Sons: 2003.
13. Holman C. Living Bereavement: An Exploration of Healthcare Workers' Responses to Loss and Grief in an NHS Continuing Care Ward for Older People. International Journal of Older People Nursing 3:278-281, 2008.

Patient-Safe Communication and Patient Education

11

Learning Outcomes

Upon completion of this chapter, you will be able to:

1. Describe the relationship among patient education, health-care literacy, and patient-safe communication.
2. Describe cognitive knowledge, affective dispositions, and psychomotor behavioral capabilities, which are the focus of teaching and learning during patient education.
3. Describe the basic assessment that must be done before teaching the patient.
4. Identify the basic components of a teaching plan.
5. Identify the major teaching methods and relate them to the content to be taught.
6. Evaluate patient learning and the effectiveness of the teaching method.

Key Words

Health-care literacy
Cognitive knowledge
Affective dispositions

Psychomotor behavioral capabilities
Principles of teaching-learning
Teaching plan

In this chapter, principles and strategies of patient-safe communication are applied to a very important nursing role responsibility: patient education. Patient-safe communication is a foundation of patient education. Health literacy is the aim of patient education. Health information can be confusing for anyone. Health literacy is "the degree to which individuals have the ability to obtain, understand and process basic health information and services needed to make appropriate health decisions."[1] Patient-safe communication is used by health professionals as they teach a patient how to obtain, understand, and process health information so that the patient is able to make informed decisions. *For an interactive version of this activity, see DavisPlus at http://davisplus.fadavis.com*

Patient-safe communication is necessary during health education for the patient to gain an understanding of health-related issues and act on health information. Low health literacy impairs the ability to navigate within the health-care environment, impairs communications between patients and health-care providers, and inadvertently leads to substandard medical care.[2-4] Patient-safe communication during health education is needed to bridge the gap between the patient's lack of ability to understand and apply health-care information and the required cognitive knowledge, affective behaviors, and psychomotor skills needed for high levels of health-care literacy.

The lack of health literacy costs billions of dollars annually in terms of health-care expenditures.[5] Millions of North Americans cannot effectively obtain, process, and understand basic health information and services needed to make informed health-care decisions and follow treatment instructions.[2-6] Low health literacy results in higher rates of disease and mortality and increased rates of hospitalization because people do not know when to seek health-care services, how to obtain needed treatments, and how to manage their health care at home effectively. For example, people with low literacy may wait too long to obtain health care when ill and then need to be hospitalized, which costs much more than had they sought care earlier and been treated in an outpatient clinic. Most patients hide their confusion because they are too intimidated or too ashamed to ask for help.[4]

To improve public health literacy, programs have been instituted through such agencies as the U.S. National Patient Safety Foundation and Canadian Manitoba Institute for Public Safety. The aim of these public programs, intended as a service for everyone living in the United States and Canada, is to teach people how to engage the services of health-care providers and learn how to interact with them. Through public media, these programs emphasize health-care providers want everyone to ask questions for their own safety, not to be intimidated or ashamed about a lack of knowledge.[7] Everyone is encouraged to ask three simple questions[8]:

1. What is my main problem?
2. What do I need to do?
3. Why is it important for me to do this?

You will need to integrate all of the communication principles and patient-safe communication strategies described in this book when educating patients for high levels of health-care literacy so that patients feel comfortable in asking questions.

NURSE AS PATIENT AND FAMILY EDUCATOR

An important role for you as a nurse is to be a patient and family educator.[9] Teaching must be focused on the very specific needs of the patient, after a careful assessment of those needs. Your patient education efforts must be firmly grounded in accepted principles of the teaching and learning process.[10-12] To teach means to impart knowledge by interacting with patients and family members using patient-safe strategies to ensure that learning can occur. Learning means that a change in cognitive knowledge, affective dispositions, or psychomotor behavioral capabilities has occurred that cannot be accounted for by biological growth. Patients thereby become health-literate.

Cognitive Knowledge

Cognitive knowledge is knowing what to do to care for oneself and how to do it. The cognitive knowledge required to change behavior includes intellectual skills and the ability to comprehend and to apply knowledge to one's lifestyle.

By telling a patient, for example, "You must reduce your cholesterol, exercise, check your blood pressure, and stop smoking," you assume that a patient has the cognitive knowledge to accomplish those goals and that the patient is sufficiently motivated to apply the knowledge to make the lifestyle changes. These assumptions can add up to a big mistake.

Affective Dispositions

Affective dispositions are the attitudes, emotions, interests, and values the patient has concerning health education that result in required changes in behavior and lifestyle. The nurse can teach the patient cognitive knowledge, but as teaching occurs the nurse must consider if the patient is motivated to make the changes and if the patient has support systems if he or she cannot perform the needed activites alone.

Psychomotor Behavioral Capabilities

Behavioral capabilities are the psychomotor skills necessary for a change to occur. There is no way to validate those capabilities without having a patient demonstrate the skill(s) he or she will be performing.

Clearly, learning is doomed to failure when a health-care provider simply tells a patient what he or she needs to do without considering the cognitive, affective, and behavioral aspects of what is required.

BASIC INFORMATION FOR PATIENTS AND FAMILIES

Most student nurses wonder where to begin teaching about a particular diagnosis and how to determine when they have covered all the essential information. There is basic information that each patient and family should know about a diagnosis and treatments. The goal is to make patients as independent as possible in providing their own care and to know when they need to seek care from their physician or nurse practitioner. Use the acronym METHOD[13,14] to remember what patients and family members need to know: medications, environment, treatments, health knowledge, outpatient/inpatient referrals, and diet. In addition to using these basic guidelines, make sure you read and critique any patient education literature you plan to give to the patient.

Medications

All patients and family caretakers need to know the names and dosages of each drug the patient must take. They must know what the drugs are for, what time the drugs should be taken, and how the drugs should be taken. They must know the common side effects of each drug and which side effects should prompt a call to the physician or nurse practitioner.

To reinforce your teaching about medications, each time you give any pill, check the patient's knowledge by asking, "What is this for?" Also ask, "When do you take this at home?" It takes only a few minutes if you plan to integrate education into whatever you are doing.

Environment

Often, a patient's environment will need to be modified to accommodate the health problem. For example, the patient's home environment might need to be modified by obtaining a portable toilet if the patient with heart problems cannot go up and down the stairs.

Take time to consider the modifications your patient's environment will need. Ensure the patient has the means to pay for whatever is needed. Many types of equipment and medications are very expensive, and some patients may not have equipment or prescription benefits in their health-care plans. You may have to teach the patient how to get financial assistance to pay for the required care. If you are not familiar with types of financial aid, then make a referral to someone in your own agency or outside agency.

Family members must be prepared to adapt as well so they do not expect too much or too little of the patient's functional abilities. Include the family in whatever teaching you give the patient whenever possible. Assess family reactions and responses just as you assess those of the patient. Family members may have to provide care for the patient and may have significant alterations in typical roles they play. If the family is not able to care for the patient at home, the patient may require home health care or placement in a long-term care facility.

Treatments

Treatments include any procedures that the patient and family must learn to do. For example, the patient may need to learn how to perform a self-injection or a self-catheterization; the family may need to change a dressing or administer oxygen. Teaching involves demonstration of how to do the procedure and always includes a return demonstration by the patient or a family member. Also included in the teaching is how to obtain supplies needed for the procedure.

Health Knowledge

The patient needs cognitive knowledge of the health problem, including important details of the disease and the signs and symptoms that require immediate attention. For example, a patient with congestive heart failure needs to know that the heart is not pumping as efficiently as it used to. To keep track of this condition, the patient should monitor weight, look for swelling in the ankles, and watch for shortness of breath and feelings of chest tightness or pain. These are all signs that the heart is not pumping efficiently.

In addition, the patient will need to know about any activity limitations created by the condition. Telling a patient, "Go home, and take it easy," is a classic educational blunder. Exactly what does "take it easy" mean? Another activity guide that is vague yet often told to patients is, "You can do only light activities." You need to be specific. Give some examples.

Exercise guidelines are very important. For example, directions include walking around in the home. Usually after major surgery or childbirth, a patient can resume (or start) a regular exercise schedule in about 6 weeks. Sexual activities must also be discussed. For example, with prostate surgery, rectovaginal surgery, or childbirth, it may take 5 to 6 weeks before it is safe to resume sexual activity to allow healing and avoid infection.

Driving is a very important activity to be discussed. For example, patients must not drive while taking pain medications that act as central nervous system depressants. Other drugs may require a period of adjustment before the patient can drive safely or operate dangerous equipment (such as an electric saw).

When the patient can return to work is also very important. Return varies with the type of exertion required on the job. In most cases, an office worker can return sooner than a laborer. In some situations, patients may need some form of occupational therapy or job retraining, and you will need to make appropriate referrals.

Outpatient/Inpatient Referrals

The patient and family must be informed about when they should be seen again by a health-care provider. In addition, the patient may need referrals to community agencies for supportive services, such as the American Heart Association, American Cancer Society, ostomy organizations, mastectomy organizations, and so on. When making referrals or telling patients about an appointment at a certain date and time, do not assume that they own a car or know how to drive. They may need a family member's help or a community transportation service.

Diet

Patients and families need to be aware of special diets to be followed. Dietary restrictions and sample menus should be provided, and they should receive counseling from a dietitian as necessary.

✚ TEACHING-LEARNING PRINCIPLES

Teaching always begins by assessing the learner.

Assess the Learner

One of the major principles of patient education is to assess the learner before beginning to teach. The assessments for patient education are based on the core and context ring of the transformational model in Chapter 2. The psycho-social-cultural assessment tool developed by Schuster (2008) in Box 11.1 can be used as a practical guide for assessing the patient.

BOX 11.1 *Psycho-Social-Cultural Assessment Tool*

1. Emotional state (mood, body language, eye contact, facial expressions)
2. Patient's life experience (previous experiences with health care)
3. Family (mood of family members; are family members supportive?)
4. Patient age (how has health problem interfered with growth and development?)
5. Relations with health-care providers (what is the patient/family level of understanding of the health problem; are they satisfied with the care given)?
6. Self-esteem and body image (changes in physical appearance; changes in activity)
7. Cultural (religious preference and practices; favorite foods; years lived in the region; travel outside the region)
8. Gender (style of speech)

Note: Information is obtained by observing verbal and nonverbal behaviors and making inferences as you and the patient work toward accomplishing objectives.

As you go into a room with teaching as your goal, always find out first what the patient's immediate mood, thoughts, and needs are; you will need to address these first. Afterward, the patient will be much more willing and able to learn. For instance, suppose you enter a patient's room and find out that she is in pain. You will need to do something to control the pain before you can start to teach. A person in pain cannot concentrate. Once you have managed basic needs and concerns, you can begin teaching by determining how well she understands the health-care problem you will be discussing. To help keep your teaching focused, you will want to ask the patient open-ended questions about the health problem she is experiencing. Allow the patient to express herself freely; doing so may give you an idea about what concerns her the most, and that will be where you need to start teaching.

Communication Safety Alert

Patients will be self-motivated to address their most urgent concerns and will tune in closely to what you are trying to teach in those areas.

Especially important is the assessment of past experiences with illness and injury. Address any misconceptions or fears the patient may have. It is especially relevant to find out about previous experiences that relate directly to the behaviors you are asking the patient to change.

Teaching methods must be selected to facilitate active participation. Learning is faster and retention is better with the active involvement of the learner. Lecturing is not appropriate because it allows no interaction, placing the learner in a dependent and passive role.[12] To teach psychomotor skills, you will need to use demonstrations. The patient becomes actively involved in giving return demonstrations to validate learning.

Communication Safety Alert

Make the patient an active participant in each teaching session. Have open discussions (not lectures) that are effective teaching strategies for cognitive and affective content. Encourage the patient to ask questions to clarify material. You should ask questions, too, to validate what the patient learned.

Assess Learning Style and Reading Level

Learning styles represent how people learn best. Questions to ask patients to try to figure out how they will learn best are as follows:

"Do you learn best by having someone go over everything point by point?"
"Would you prefer to watch a video, listen to an audiotape, use a computerized learning program, or read by yourself first and then ask questions?"
"Can you hear and see me okay?"

Communication Safety Alert

With a patient who is sight-impaired, large-size print materials or audiotapes might work best. With a patient who cannot hear, printed materials and videotapes with subtitles can be useful. With patients who have hearing impairments, speak slowly and distinctly, and ask them to repeat frequently to make sure they have heard what you said. Sometimes it may look as if a person is hearing you, but if you ask the person to repeat, the person cannot.

A prime consideration is the patient's reading level. Many patients who are illiterate may be too embarrassed to admit it. One of five adults reads at a fifth-grade level or lower. A tactful way to evaluate reading is to ask, "Do you like to read?" If the answer is no, you will need to find another way to present the information without embarrassing the person. If the patient wears glasses, does he or she have them on? Most people older than 40 have special glasses for reading. Although there is patient teaching literature readily available on almost any topic, you must evaluate first whether the patient can read it and then comprehend and apply it to his or her personal situation.

Assess Readiness to Learn

You will also need to determine whether the patient is ready, willing, and able to learn. If the person is in pain, tired, hungry, anxious, fearful, in denial, or distracted, you are wasting time by trying to teach; learning will not take place.

Say, for example, that a patient came up from the cardiac catheterization lab around noon. The patient was tired after being in the lab for about 3 hours for testing. The patient was also hungry because he was not allowed to eat before the test and lunch had not yet been delivered. The patient also was uncomfortable because he had to stay in bed and lie still with a pressure dressing and sandbag on the leg that had been catheterized. At that point, the dietitian walked in, pulled up a chair, and started teaching him about a low-fat, low-salt cardiac diet. How much do you imagine the patient learned about the diet? Probably nothing. If the health-care provider had assessed the patient first and applied basic principles of teaching, he would have known to leave this patient alone until he had eaten and rested. The patient was polite and said nothing, although some patients might have said, "I'm tired, hungry, and uncomfortable. Can you come back later when I can actually hear what you're trying to tell me?" Even if the patient does not speak, you will have clues to learning readiness. If at any point during a teaching session, a patient's eyes glaze over, you have lost that patient.

You can make the most of your time and the patient's time by incorporating teaching into your ongoing patient care. Each time you are with a patient, you can teach and validate what has been taught before. As you change a dressing, you can discuss wound care or signs and symptoms of infection. Take action at every teachable moment. In addition, keep the time between learning the information and applying the information as short as possible to help the patient retain the information.

You can also make the most of your time by involving the patient's family in the teaching. Have family members present whenever possible. They can reinforce instructions.

Assess Patient Financial Status

You must know how much the drugs, dressings, or other needed supplies will cost the patient, whether the patient's health plan covers them, and whether the patient can afford what is left over (out of pocket) after the insurance is finished.

Assess Family Support Systems

What family and friends are available to the patient? Are they supportive of the patient emotionally? Do they agree that the treatments are appropriate? Ask, "How has the illness affected your family?"

After Assessment

It is important after assessing and teaching to reinforce learning and to solicit feedback.

Reinforce All Learning

It is crucial that you remember to give positive reinforcement each time the patient takes a step toward making a change—even a small step. Document your teaching and the patient's progress. Communicate your progress with patient teaching to other health-care professionals who will care for the patient. Share information about what the patient has learned and what still requires more teaching and reinforcement. Let your colleagues know which teaching methods were and were not effective for this patient. You may also want to refer a patient to a support group for ongoing help with making needed changes, reinforcing behaviors, and maintaining behavior changes.

Solicit Feedback

In the case of patient education, the feedback is in the form of evaluating what the patient has learned. Just because you go over information with someone, you cannot assume the person knows what you mean or knows how to do what you asked.

Start an evaluation by asking if the patient has any questions after you present information or finish your discussion. After you address these questions, ask some additional questions to confirm the patient's understanding. Ask the patient to restate information, for example, "Let's review a little bit so I know that I clearly explained the signs of bladder infection to you. Can you tell me what signs you should watch for that might mean you have an infection in your bladder?"

Another excellent way to find out what a patient has learned is by making up a brief scenario that relates to the patient's life and then asking how the patient would handle it. You can evaluate both cognitive and affective forms of learning with oral questions. Return demonstrations are the only way to evaluate performance of a psychomotor skill.

FACTORS THAT INHIBIT LEARNING

Nurses must keep in mind several factors that can inhibit learning. When these factors are present, they must be under control before learning can occur.

Emotions

You should recognize and empathize with emotions when working with a patient. Evaluate the patient's emotional state first before teaching or doing anything else. Emotions are a prime consideration as you communicate, either when teaching or attempting any other form of communication. For example, if the patient is extremely anxious, you need to reduce anxiety prior to attempting teaching.

Defense Mechanisms

A patient who is in denial about an illness or rationalizing about why he or she cannot do something will need to get beyond that point before any behavioral changes can be made.

Physiological Problems

A patient's physiological state can interfere with learning also. When someone is tired, hungry, in pain, nauseated, or vomiting, you will need to postpone your lesson until the physiological problem has been resolved.

Cultural Barriers

Often, patients and family members have values that differ from yours and those of other health-care providers. For example, say you explain to an Amish man that he needs an electric implanted defibrillator to control his heart arrhythmia or he will die. Amish people do not have electricity in their homes, and they believe modern conveniences are "the work of the devil." This patient may choose to die rather than have an electrical device implanted in his body.

Sometimes you will need to accept a patient's beliefs and avoid trying to impose the values of the medical community on him. All teaching is geared toward the lifestyle of the patient, which includes the patient's culture.

Special Considerations of Patient Education With Children

All that has been said about teaching adults applies to teaching children as well. You must always include the parents, and obtain their cooperation in your teaching. You will need to take the child's stage of cognitive development into consideration.

MAJOR COMPONENTS OF A TEACHING PLAN

Now that you know generally what you are supposed to be teaching and how to do a basic assessment, you need to develop a plan with specific goals and objectives, with teaching methods for each goal and objective. The plan has to be individualized to what you assessed about the patient.

Assessment

Suppose you have assessed that a patient has a knowledge deficit about his newly diagnosed diabetes and the need to take insulin. He first wants to learn about insulin and how to give his own injections. He is 55 years old, has a college degree, has been an investment broker for the past 25 years, and wants to get back to work as soon as possible. He is motivated to learn, he likes to read, and his family is supportive. His wife wants to attend nutrition classes to learn the new diet and how to modify the way she currently cooks. The patient's insurance plan covers prescription medications and the supplies needed for injecting insulin.

Goals and Objectives

Based on this assessment, the general goal will be to have the patient self-administer insulin. Tailor the information you present so the goals are attainable by the patient you are teaching. Remember that the average adult can remember only five to seven things at a time, so keep your teachings short, simple, and specific. The more information you present, the more the patient will forget. Less information is really more, because the information will be better retained. Never try to present everything in one teaching session. Teaching small amounts of information over time is much more effective.[15]

Write specific objectives to address cognitive, affective, and psychomotor learning behaviors that the patient must attain to meet the goal successfully.

Cognitive learning objectives specify that the patient do the following:

- Describe the purpose of insulin
- Describe the adverse effects of too much or too little insulin
- State what to do if side effects occur

Affective learning objectives specify that the patient do the following:

- Listen to instructions on how to perform self-injection
- State that an injection is necessary and why it is necessary
- Show no signs of anxiety and appear relaxed

Psychomotor learning objectives specify the patient do the following:

- Assemble supplies needed to self-administer insulin
- Draw into the syringe the correct dosage of the drug without contaminating the equipment
- Inject insulin without contaminating the needle

Note that all these objectives are clearly measurable.

Teaching Strategies

Next, you must plan the teaching strategies that will meet the objectives. The strategies discussed in the following sections are grouped according to whether learning objectives are cognitive, affective, or psychomotor.

Cognitive Objectives

Cognitive knowledge is usually taught using printed and audiovisual materials. These include books, pamphlets, films, programmed instruction, and computer learning. Learners can proceed at their own pace, and the nurse does not need to be present during learning.

Cognitive knowledge can also be learned when you give explanations and descriptions in a lecture to the patient and family members. You control the content and the pace of the instruction; however, the learner is passive and will retain less information than when being an active participant in the learning process.

In addition, cognitive knowledge may be gained by encouraging the patient to ask questions. Confirm that each question has been answered by asking the learner, "Does that answer your question?"

Affective and Cognitive Objectives

Affective and cognitive knowledge can be gained from one-to-one discussion that permits the introduction of sensitive issues and encourages participation by the learner. You can provide immediate reinforcement and as much repetition as needed until the patient learns the objectives of the lesson. Group discussions may also be useful to attain affective and cognitive objectives when the members support each other, share their ideas and concerns, and problem-solve together.

Role playing is a teaching strategy that encourages the expression of attitudes, values, and emotions, and it allows active involvement by the learner. In addition, affective and cognitive behaviors may be learned by the teaching strategy of discovery, which involves guiding the patient through practice situations requiring the patient to solve problems surrounding the diagnosis or treatments. When the patient is an active participant, the retention of information is higher.

Psychomotor Objectives

Psychomotor skills are taught by demonstrations accompanied by explanations. You must give very clear and specific directions, and show patients what they must do. Demonstrations must be accompanied by the teaching strategy of guided practice. The patient must have "hands-on" experience, with repetition and immediate feedback from you.

Implementation of Teaching

After developing the plan, it is now time for patient-nurse interaction. Make sure to choose a good time for the interaction. A good time might be after breakfast, after the patient has slept well, when the patient has no discomforts and is ready to learn. This environment is optimal.

Order the learning activities by starting with the basics. For example, you are teaching the patient to self-administer insulin subcutaneously. Give the patient pamphlets, and tell the patient that you will return in an hour to talk about questions. When you return, answer the questions, and have a one-to-one discussion regarding affective behaviors. Next, take the patient to a small classroom where the movie and equipment are prepared ahead of time. Play the movie, give a live demonstration, and follow this up with practice by the patient on a mannequin. Last, have the patient self-inject insulin the next time it is due to be given. In addition, use simple everyday language, avoiding medical terminology whenever possible. There is a big difference between saying "Let's talk about hypoglycemia and signs and symptoms of insulin shock" and saying "Let's talk about what to do when you have low blood sugar and feel shaky or light-headed."

Evaluation and Documentation of Learning and Teaching

The last step in the teaching and learning process is to evaluate whether learning occurred and if the teaching methods were effective and to document what was done. In order to evaluate, ask yourself, "Did the patient learn about insulin and how to give the injection?" More specifically, ask yourself, "Did the patient master each of the objectives?"

You must specifically evaluate each objective. Typically, cognitive objectives can be evaluated by giving the patient a test, oral or written. Affective behaviors can be inferred from how the patient responds to questions and speaks about relevant topics. In addition, you can observe behaviors that express feelings and values. Psychomotor behavior is measured by direct observation. The patient may be able to describe each step in the procedure, and you must see the patient perform the activity to validate a psychomotor skill.

To continue with the example of the diabetic patient, you will evaluate cognitive knowledge by asking questions and giving the patient examples of situations for which he would describe his response. For example, "You're driving in your car about 11 a.m. after giving yourself insulin at 8 a.m. You become light-headed, you start sweating, and you feel shaky. What do you think is wrong, and what should you do?" Next, you evaluate the patient's psychomotor abilities by telling him to pretend that you are not there and to do everything needed to draw up and administer the injection just as he will be doing at home. In addition, you evaluate his affective behaviors by noting how he responds to your questions and how his facial expressions change as he gives himself an injection. You evaluate psychomotor skills by watching the patient give his own injection.

Communication Safety Alert

You will never know for sure that a patient has learned what is required unless you evaluate the patient's learning by asking questions regarding cognitive knowledge, noting the affective response and motivational levels, and asking for a return demonstration for psychomotor skills.

Last is the evaluation of your teaching methods. Was the timing of your teaching appropriate? Were your strategies effective? Was the amount of information appropriate? You can ask your patient for insight either verbally or in writing. By evaluating oral or written responses, you can tell whether your objectives were met. Other characteristics of effective teaching include the ability to hold the patient's interest and the ability to make the patient a partner—an active participant—in the teaching and learning process. Good teachers are also optimistic, positive, nonthreatening, and supportive of a positive self-concept in learners. They help patients believe they can accomplish all objectives. Good teachers typically use several methods of teaching that are appropriate for the objectives and the learning style of the patient.

CHAPTER SUMMARY

This chapter describes basic principles of teaching and learning required for effective patient education. The nurse develops patient educational objectives that are focused on the cognitive knowledge, affective dispositions, and behavioral capabilities pertaining to the patient's specific health state and required knowledge needed for self-care. Knowledge of how to perform a learning assessment, develop a teaching plan, implement teaching, and evaluate learning are essential patient-safe strategies to educate patients and families using high-level communication competency. Also, it is important to evaluate the effectiveness of the teaching strategies and then modify teaching strategies as needed for patients and families to attain learning outcomes. Health literacy is the intended result of patient education.

 BUILDING HIGH-LEVEL COMMUNICATION COMPETENCE

For additional exercises, see DavisPlus at http://davisplus.fadavis.com

1. **Patient Education Practice and Critical Thinking.** The following three patients are newly diagnosed with diabetes and require insulin to control the disease. The nurse must teach each of the three patients about administering insulin to themselves safely. Each has a special learning need. For each patient, address the following three questions: What other assessment data would you like to know about the patient? What patient-safe strategies would you use to obtain the needed assessment information? How would you customize the goals, objectives, teaching strategies, and evaluation methods for each patient?
   Patient 1 is legally blind.
   Patient 2 has been up all night because of a noisy roommate and feels very tired.
   Patient 3 exclaims, "I get queasy and feel like fainting whenever I look at that needle!"

2. **Critical Thinking.** Amanda Severt is 35 years old and is being treated for an overactive thyroid. Your assessment reveals that she is weak and tired and has lost 30 pounds. She is 5'6" and weighs 110 pounds, even though she eats an enormous amount of food. She is taking medication, but you would like to teach her about increasing her calorie intake to gain weight. You are to provide nutritional teaching. Where do you start?

3. **Communication Practice.** As a class activity to practice patient-safe strategies and patient teaching, role-play the above-mentioned situations in front of the class. One student can be the nurse, the other student can be the patient, and the interaction can be evaluated by the entire class.

References

1. Healthy People 2010. Washington, D.C., U.S. Department of Health and Human Services, Office of Disease Prevention and Health Promotion.
2. Berkman, N.D., DeWalt, D.A., Pignone, M.P., et al. Literacy and Health Outcomes: Summary, Evidence Report, Technology Assessment, number 87. AHRQ Publication Number 04-E007-1. Rockville, Md., Agency for Healthcare Research and Quality: January 2004. Located at http://www.ahrq.gov/clinic/epcsums/litsum.htm Accessed January, 2009.
3. Schwartzberg, J.G., VanGeest, J.B., Wang, C.C. (eds.). Understanding Health Literacy: Implications for Medicine and Public Health. Atlanta, American Medical Association Press: 2005.

4. Abrams, M., American Medical Association. Health Literacy and Patient Safety: Help Patients Understand: Removing Barriers to Better, Safer Care: Reducing the Risk by Designing a Safer, Shame-Free Healthcare Environment. Atlanta, American Medical Association Press: 2007.
5. Potter, L., Martin, C. Health Literacy Fact Sheets. Center for Healthcare Strategies: 2005. Located at http://www.chcs.org/publications3960/publications_show.htm?doc_id=291711 Accessed January, 2009.
6. Canadian Public Health Association. National Literacy and Health Program. Located at http://www.nlhp.cpha.ca/ Accessed January, 2009.
7. Manitoba Institute for Public Safety. It's Safe to Ask. Located at http://www.safetoask.ca/ Accessed January, 2009.
8. Partnership for Clear Health Communication at the National Patient Safety Foundation. Ask Me 3. Located at http://www.npsf.org/askme3/ Accessed January, 2009.
9. DeYoung, S. Teaching Strategies for Nurse Educators, 2nd ed. Upper Saddle River, N.J., Pearson/ Prentice-Hall: 2009.
10. Knowles, M.S. The Modern Practice of Adult Education: From Pedagogy to Androgogy. Wilton, Conn., Association Press: 1980.
11. Knowles, M.S., Holton, E.F., Swanson, R.A. The Adult Learner: The Definitive Classic in Adult Education and Human Resource Development, 6th ed. Burlington, Mass., Elsevier: 2005.
12. Bastable, S.B. Nurse as Educator: Principles of Teaching and Learning for Nursing Practice. Sudbury, Mass., Jones and Bartlett: 2008.
13. Huey, R. Discharge Planning: Good Planning Means Fewer Hospitalizations for the Chronically Ill. Nursing 81:11–20, 1981.
14. Schuster, P.M. Concept Mapping: A Critical-Thinking Apprach to Care Planning, 2nd ed. Philadelphia, FA Davis: 2008.
15. Willingham, D.T. Practice Makes Perfect—But Only If You Practice Beyond the Point of Perfection. American Educator 38:31-33, 2004.

3

Health-Care Team Communication: Group Processes and Patient-Safe Communication Among Team Members

Patient Safety Communication Risk Factors in Nursing Work Systems

Learning Outcomes

Upon completion of this chapter, you will be able to:

1. Describe the communication responsibilities of the nurse in promoting patient safety during communication with other members of the health-care team.
2. Compare the person approach and systems approach to human errors in health-care systems.
3. Relate human cognition and performance to mental antecedents of human error involving errors of execution, errors of decision making, and deliberate violations of rules.
4. Describe the relationship among performance inputs, process, and outputs of the nursing work system.
5. Using accident causation theory, describe how patient care errors occur.
6. Describe conditions in the work environment of nursing work systems that create communication failures and harmful events.

Key Terms

Patient monitoring
Coordination of care
Continuity in care
Care transitions
Human factors
Human strengths
Human limitations
Human error
Error
Automatic mode
Mixed mode
Conscious mode
Error of execution
Error of decision making
Skill-based error
Rule-based error
Knowledge-based error

Slips
Lapses
Mistakes
Violations
Mental model
Situational awareness
Working memory
System
Systems perspective
Performance inputs
Process
Performance outputs
Active failure
Latent condition
Error-provoking conditions
Person approach
Systems approach

The purpose of this chapter is to describe the characteristics of patient safety communication risk factors encountered during intradisciplinary (nurse-nurse) communications and interdisciplinary (nurse–other discipline) communications within nursing work systems. Over the past decade, communication failures between health-care team members have become widely recognized as a leading safety hazard in health care,[1] hampering the ability to deliver safe, high-quality care. This chapter explores the growing evidence that factors in the health-care system and nursing work environment are the major contributors to communication failures between members of the health-care team. From this broad perspective, nurses can learn how communication failures happen, recognize risks for communication failure in their work environment, use patient-safe communication strategies specific to working with members of the health-care team, and advocate for health-care system improvements to keep patients safe. Review Figure 2.5, and identify communication risk factors involving intradisciplinary and interdisciplinary communications in the Transformational Model of Communication.

Nurses represent the largest discipline within the health-care workforce and provide the greatest amount of direct patient care and integration of patient care services across the professions. They are uniquely positioned to communicate essential patient information with other members of the health-care team.

COMMUNICATION OF ESSENTIAL PATIENT INFORMATION

Primary activities within the role of the nurse that involve communicating essential patient information to other health-care team members include patient monitoring, coordination of care, and maintaining continuity in care.

Patient Monitoring

A primary activity and role of nurses is ongoing patient monitoring. Patient monitoring is the ongoing assessment and evaluation of patient health status and involves the purposeful acquisition, interpretation, and synthesis of patient information for clinical decision making.[2] It is an important surveillance mechanism for detecting errors, detecting early deterioration of patient health status, and preventing harmful events.[3] Performance of patient monitoring requires great attention, knowledge, and responsiveness on the part of the nurse,[3] and the findings must be carefully communicated orally to other team members and documented on patient records. With the early recognition and effective communication of the deterioration in patient health status, there is rapid initiation of coordinated activities to restore patient health.

Coordination of Care

In addition to monitoring patients, nurses serve as the coordinator or integrator of patient care and services from multiple members of the health-care team. Nurses coordinate the scheduling and implementation of all treatments and therapies of physicians, pharmacists, dietitians, social workers, and other members of the health-care team. Updates in patient health status from incoming information, such as laboratory results, or changes in the treatment plans are communicated by nurses as appropriate. Nurses review patient records to detect gaps in information and take action to implement changes in treatment plans through communication with other health-care team members. Failure to communicate timely and accurate treatment updates during coordination of care results in treatment delays and can jeopardize patient health.[4]

Maintaining Continuity of Care During Care Transitions

Nurses also serve a role in maintaining continuity of care during care transitions, defined as patient transfers from one care provider to another (for example, from one nurse to another or from one care setting to another, such as from a hospital to a community care setting).[5,6] During care transitions, nurses maintain continuity of care by communicating patient status, plan of care, and any anticipated changes to watch for in the next interval of care.[7] By means of patient monitoring, coordination of care, and maintaining continuity in care, nurses and nursing communications are inseparably linked to patient safety and prevention of harmful events.

The Person Approach Versus the Systems Approach to Patient Care Errors

The Institute of Medicine (IOM) report, "To Err is Human—Building a Safer Health System"[8] reported that health care is not as safe as it should be and described tens of thousands of people who die annually from medical errors in hospitals. Analyses of over 2000 medical errors revealed that 70% was the result of communication failure and, of these, approximately 75% of patients died.[9]

One of the main conclusions from the IOM report was that the majority of errors in health care was the result of faulty systems, processes, and conditions that led individuals to make mistakes rather than the result of individual recklessness.[8] "People working in healthcare are among the most dedicated workforce in any industry. The problem is not bad people; the problem is that the system needs to be made safer."[10]

The IOM claimed that the focus must shift from blaming individuals for patient care errors (person approach) to a focus on preventing future errors by designing safety into the health-care system at all levels (systems approach). The IOM opened the door for health-care team members and organizational leaders to understand errors as a symptom of an unsafe system. Viewing errors from a "systems" perspective takes into consideration how factors within the system itself affect human performance, which can lead to patient care errors.

Improving safety from a systems perspective is important because no matter where you choose to work, you will be working within a system that has safety issues. Trying to be more careful and more cautious will do little if safety issues in the system remain unresolved.[10] By understanding the systems approach taken by the IOM, you will have a broader focus both on identifying the underlying safety issues and recommending improvements for safety that address these issues. Implementing change through a systems perspective, rather than reacting to errors as they occur, is the only way far-reaching quality improvements in safety can be achieved.[10]

Competencies for health-care team members related to systems thinking and patient safety include but are not limited to[11]:

- Understanding system design and its impact on safety
- Risk awareness through anticipating and recognizing problems at the level of individuals and of systems
- Correcting safety issues to prevent them from reaching the patient

Collectively, the competencies afford nurses and other team members with opportunities to help build a safer health-care system. To attain these competencies, health-care providers need to examine the relationships among people, job performance requirements, and the work environment using a human factors science theoretical perspective. Human factors science is the study of the fit between the tasks that people do and the work environment.

Human Factors Science

The science of human factors is about "goodness of fit": the fit between people, the things they do, the objects they use, and the environments they work in.[12] If a good fit is achieved, it reduces the stresses on people. They are more comfortable, they can do things more easily and, most important, they make fewer mistakes. Human factors science involves the design of an interactive work system that ensures the effectiveness, safety, and ease of use of tools and equipment and effective performance of tasks by workers within the work environment.[13] For nurses, this means that the tasks they perform, the tools they use, the work environment in which they function, and the organizational policies that shape their activities must be designed to be a good fit for their human abilities and limitations.[14]

When system factors and human sensory, cognitive, and behavioral abilities are poorly matched, substandard outcomes frequently occur in quality of care and patient safety.[3,14] A thorough understanding of human abilities and limitations that affect performance is essential to understanding how a work system must be designed.

✜ HUMAN ABILITIES AND LIMITATIONS AFFECTING PERFORMANCE

By their very nature, humans make errors.[15] In any industry, one of the greatest contributors to accidents or harmful events is human error. It has been estimated that human error is the cause of up to 90% of all organizational accidents.[16] In health care, 70% to 82% of incidents analyzed in the operating room have been attributed to human error.[17,18] Keep in mind, however, that saying an incident or harmful event is due to human error is not the same as assigning blame.[10] Humans are fallible and make errors for a variety of reasons that have little to do with lack of good intention or knowledge.[19] Difficulty in maintaining continual alertness, inability to attend to several things at once, having habits of thought and action, and lacking precision in mental functioning are our human weaknesses.

Human error is the category of human performance that leads to bad outcomes.[20] James Reason, a British psychologist and expert on human factors science, defines human error as the failure of a planned action to achieve its intended goal.[21] Human errors involve cognitive processes of mental functioning as people plan actions and yet fail in their attempts to reach intended outcomes. Human errors are directly related to cognitive human performance. For example, a nurse may become cognitively impaired from fatigue, leading to human errors when she is mandated to work a double shift, and she is expected to perform mathematical calculations involving the administration of medications. When this nurse makes a medication calculation error, it is due to cognitive impairments as a result of fatigue stemming from the hospital policy of mandatory overtime.

Investigations into major industrial accidents have increased understanding of human cognitive performance in the work environment. There is evidence-based knowledge of why people err, and a great deal has been learned about how to design work environments to minimize the occurrence of errors and limit their consequences.[22,23] The study of how human errors occur has led to the development of normal cognition theory to explain how humans think during the performance of activities.

Normal Cognition Theory

During performance of activities, Reason describes normal human cognition as involving three modes—automatic, conscious, and mixed. Characteristics of each are as follows[21]:

Automatic Mode

Most of your thinking during the performance of activities operates in the automatic mode. We use the automatic mode during often-repeated, routine tasks. The automatic mode is associated with our long-term memory. Long-term memory has unlimited capacity and can process parallel bits of information simultaneously rather than process one thing after the other. For example, you can leave home, drive to the campus, park, and go to your classroom without devoting much conscious thought to any of the hundreds of maneuvers and decisions that this complex set of activities requires.

Automatic processing is possible because you carry a vast array of mental models in your long-term memory that store the many recurrent aspects of everyday life. Your cognitive mental models are essential for you to function in our environment, and they operate quickly, processing information rapidly and without conscious effort.

Conscious Mode

You use conscious critical thinking processing when you are in a new situation that does not match any of our mental models, and you have a problem to solve. The problem is worked out through purposeful critical thinking. The conscious mode entails the use of short-term working memory. Working memory can only process one thing at a time and is difficult to maintain because conscious critical thought requires our full attention to what we are doing. People have a limited ability to focus their attention on more than one thing at a time when they have the need to be operating in the conscious mode. As an example of conscious mode and working memory, remember when you first got behind the wheel of the car, or you were learning to take a blood pressure or insert a urinary catheter. You had to concentrate and think purposefully as you studied books, viewed movies, and practiced performing the skills for many hours before doing these things on your own.

Human attention to a task that requires critical thinking can be sustained only for fairly short periods, usually about 20 minutes, after which fatigue sets in. Additionally, when attention is focused on one thing, it is necessarily withdrawn from all other things.[24,25] In sum, working memory critical thinking processing is slow, sequential, takes effort, is limited in capacity, and requires full conscious attention.

Mixed Mode

Somewhere in between operating automatically and consciously is a mixed control mode. You use this when you encounter a trained-for situation. Here, you need to modify our largely programmed automatic behaviors because you need to take into account some change in the situation or procedure. You apply memorized rules when automatically matching the signs and symptoms of the problem to some stored mental model; you also operate consciously to verify whether the solution is appropriate. For example, you may be proficient at taking a blood pressure and can perform the psychomotor task automatically. You will have to operate in conscious mode as well, however, when you encounter a patient who is very thin with severe contractures, making it difficult for you to hear her blood pressure using an adult cuff. There is no pediatric cuff available, and you remember that you could perform a palpation blood pressure. You consciously verify the solution is appropriate because the patient has good pulses. You had to develop a new rule for how to take a blood pressure when a patient has contractures. You can then apply this new rule when you encounter this situation in the future. You have added to your mental model of how to obtain a blood pressure.

How Error Occurs

There are two ways to make an error. Reason[21,25-27] describes errors of execution and errors in decision making; these result in the failure of a planned action to achieve its intended goal.

- **Error of execution:** The plan is adequate but does not proceed as intended.
- **Error in decision making:** A wrong plan is used to achieve an aim.

Errors of Execution

Errors of execution happen during the largely automatic performance of a routine, often-repeated task. These errors occur at the skill-based level of human performance and are further divided into two groups: slips and lapses. Slips are associated with attention failure, and lapses are associated with memory failure. Highly practiced and automatic behaviors are particularly susceptible to attention and memory failures. Attention and memory failures are typically caused by internal preoccupation, daydreaming, or being in a hurry. Distractions in the immediate surroundings can shift attention away from the task at hand and cause a slip; interruptions can cause you to forget to do something and cause a lapse.

A variety of internal factors can make slips and lapses more likely. Physiological factors include physical fatigue, alcohol, drugs, and illness. Psychological factors include emotional states such as boredom, frustration, fear, stress, panic, mental fatigue, anxiety, and anger. Each of these factors leads to preoccupation, which diverts attention from the task at hand.

Memory failures (lapses) can cause a nurse to forget essential details of patient information, which, for example, can result in forgetting to pass on important information at change-of-shift report. Memory failures can also result in items omitted from a preoperative checklist or nursing admission database.[15]

Errors in Decision Making

Errors in decision making happen during the conscious performance of problem solving in trained-for and novel situations. Errors in decision making occur at the higher rule-based and knowledge-based cognitive level of human performance. They are associated with perception failures, misinterpretations, and lack of essential information. Errors in decision making are called "honest mistakes"[15] and can be divided into two groups:

Rule-based mistakes: People are very good at pattern matching and can make rapid assessments of situations based on matching features of a current situation to those stored in long-term memory. But individuals can apply the wrong rule to a patient situation (if X, then do Y) if they fail to notice contradictions, especially if there is missing or ambiguous information. The presumption results in misperception of the patient's deteriorating clinical situation. In a rule-based mistake, the nurse may, for example, implement a "wait and see" intervention rather than rapidly initiate communication coordinating activities to restore patient health.

Knowledge-based mistakes: Knowledge-based mistakes occur because of lack of knowledge, information, or misinterpretation of the problem. Individuals do not have a mental model or automatic solution in long-term memory. They have to develop a mental model of the current situation, which is nearly always incomplete. Certain habits of thought alter conscious reasoning and contribute to this process. One such process is biased memory, in that individuals perceive by what they know. They interpret novel situations within this biased framework. Recall from perception theory in Chapter 3 that people cannot experience the world directly; rather, they interpret it. Therefore, in new situations, health-care providers interpret the patient situation only by what they already know.

Another process of knowledge-based mistakes is the tendency to "fixate" on a particular guess or hunch about what is occurring in a situation. This is known as confirmation bias, described by Sir Francis Bacon more than 300 years ago.[28] With confirmation bias, individuals have the tendency to look for evidence that supports what they believe to be occurring and supports their "hunch" and ignore information that contradicts it. Health-care providers will "see" the information they expect that confirms their expectations, rather than see the information that is actually present that contradicts what they expect.[29] Knowledge-based errors can manifest the same way as rule-based errors, with delays in communicating changes in patient clinical status quickly and effectively or as inaccurate interpretations of patient information shared with other health-care team members.

Communication Safety Alert

The human mind has inherent limitations in mental functioning. Being aware of your mind's vulnerability to stress and time pressures as well as long hours and fatigue can help you recognize when you may be at risk for error.

Violations

Violations are deliberate deviations from standard practices, policies, and procedures.[27] People purposely break rules when there are poor operating procedures, inadequate work environments, low morale, time pressures, and tools and equipment that cause frustration. Routine violations occur habitually in health care. They include behaviors such as cutting corners or bending the rules to get the job done on time. Routine violations continue to be committed in the absence of incidents and are tolerated by management.[27]

Health-care team members are creative and often respond to a system problem with a "quick fix," or break from standard procedure. The immediate problem is solved but the underlying problems are ignored and allowed to continue.[30] In a recent study that examined human factors in a cardiovascular operating room, nurses stated that they were more prone to break the rules when they were rushed.[31] Conditions that created a rushed work environment for the nurses included overbooking of the operating room with subsequent overtime hours and understaffing. The nurses indicated that they would break the rules only when there was no perceived impact on patient outcome.

Violations can set in gradually over time and become the accepted norm of work behavior. Violations can become so routine and so common as to be almost invisible to both workers and management, reflective of the "fish and water" effect discussed in Chapter 3. In her investigation of the Challenger accident, in which moments after liftoff the space shuttle exploded, killing all seven astronauts, Diane Vaughan[32] discovered how gradual departures from safety became accepted as normal. She referred to this organizational behavior as normalization of deviance. In the days preceding the Challenger launch, individuals tried, unsuccessfully, to bring attention to safety concerns about the mission. The concerns were dismissed as "acceptable risk." Over time, normalization of deviance, when combined with other factors, creates thin margins of safety in an organization; in this case, it ultimately led to disaster.[32]

THE NURSING WORK SYSTEM

In the health-care system, nurses are one of many interdependent components that interact to achieve the common goal of safe, high-quality patient care and optimal patient health outcomes. A general definition of a system is a set of interdependent components that interact to achieve a common goal.[14] The interdependent components of the health-care system include nurses, patients, other health-care providers, administrators, and support staff and the patient-safe communication strategies and other tools nurses use in the health-care system.

Nurses interact on a daily basis with many components at different levels of the health-care system. From a systems perspective, the focus is on the interdependencies and interactions among the components, not on the components themselves.[14] The levels can be considered in two ways.

First, they are levels of a hierarchy. For example, the vice president of nursing is above several directors of nursing, who are above unit managers, who are above charge nurses, who are above staff nurses.[33] Each higher and broader level of a system provides context for the systems nested beneath it. The context includes policies and procedures, norms, technologies, physical environment, and people.[34,35]

Second, levels exert influence on the levels below and above, with impacts on individuals, groups, or the organization.[14,21,36] Norms, policies, and decisions at the group and organizational level affect individuals. Similarly, individual decisions can influence outcomes at the group or organization level. Policies and procedures made at a high organizational level affect groups and individuals at other levels nested beneath.[37]

Often, decisions made at higher system levels can exert influence on other levels in ways that can unexpectedly contribute to work conditions that lead to human error. This is because it is difficult in complex organizations to predict how system components across levels will interact, especially when changes are introduced.[21] If health-care providers re-examine the decisions made at a higher organizational level to improve handoff, this seemingly good change can certainly improve patient information transfer. If the new procedure is confusing or difficult to work with, however, and training has been inadequate, it may decrease the nurses' availability to conduct timely communications with physicians about patient concerns, which in turn affects the safety of patients. The point to bear in mind is that changes in one part of the system will always have effects on another part of the system.[21] This is a dynamic characteristic of all complex systems, especially the nursing work system.

A Concept Map of the Nursing Work System

Figure 12.1 illustrates a nursing work system concept map the authors have developed from the perspective of human factors science. It has been adapted from the frameworks developed by Vincent,[38] Henriksen,[14] Karsh,[35] and Carayon.[34] The concept map does not represent the full breadth of a nursing work system; rather, it focuses on a variety of systems factors known to influence nursing performance in monitoring patients, coordinating care, maintaining continuity in care, and communicating effectively face to face, over the phone, and in writing with other health-care providers.

There are three main areas in the concept map:

1. Performance Inputs, which guide the nursing work system
2. Process the required human performance to change inputs into outputs
3. Performance Outputs, the outcome of the inputs and process

A full discussion of this concept map can be found at *DavisPlus* at *http://davisplus. fadavis.com*

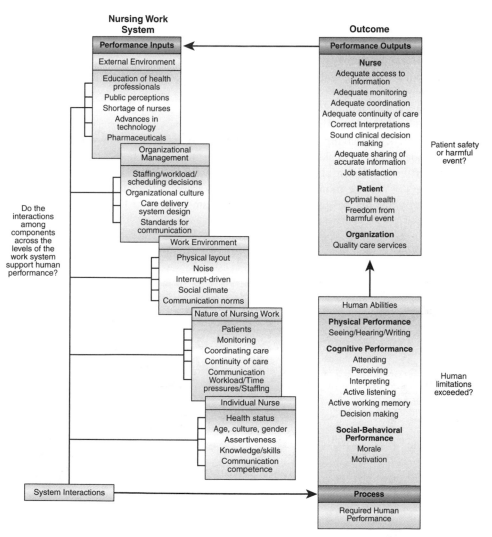

Figure 12.1 Nursing Work System.

The Nursing Work System concept map illustrates how system inputs can influence nurses' ability to perform their work activities and how that ability affects patient outcomes. Just as a well-functioning work system can facilitate performance, a poorly functioning work system can create the conditions that lead to human error, communication failures, and harmful events.[39]

Next is a discussion of how system factors create hazardous conditions that facilitate human errors, using James Reason's accident causation theory.

ACCIDENT CAUSATION THEORY

James Reason's accident causation theory provides the necessary framework to guide critical thinking in nursing about system influences on human performance that can lead to human error, communication failures, and harmful events. Reason's accident causation model[40] has been used to explain that when system components across levels are functioning well together, they serve collectively as a barrier or system of defenses to the occurrence of harmful events. Defenses to prevent the occurrence of harmful events include adequate staffing and appropriate workload. When weaknesses or vulnerabilities exist, such as inadequate staffing and heavy workload, they interact in such a way that the barriers of system defenses are breached, and harmful events occur.

Organizational system defenses occupy key positions in a health-care system to safeguard against hazards that cause harmful events. Defenses have been characterized as slices of Swiss cheese, having many holes.[40] Unlike Swiss cheese, however, these holes continually open, close, and shift their location. The presence of holes does not normally cause a harmful event. Harmful events happen only when holes in many successive system levels or layers of defense momentarily line up and propel a trajectory of error and accident opportunity that reaches patients. This is illustrated in Figure 12.2.

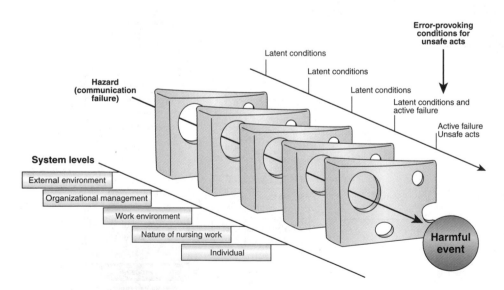

Accident trajectory penetrates successive layers of system defenses

Figure 12.2 Model of the "Swiss cheese" Nursing Work System.

Reason[40] states that holes in the defenses arise for two reasons: active failure and latent conditions. Nearly all harmful events within the nursing work system involve a combination of active failures and latent conditions.

Active Failures
Active failures are the unsafe acts committed by nurses, physicians, and other health-care providers.[40] Unsafe acts are human errors, including attention slips, memory lapses, and honest mistakes, as well as intentional violations. Reason describes these individuals as being on the "sharp end" of occurrences, as their acts have an immediate effect on patient safety. Most often, health-care administrators look no further for the cause of the harmful event once they have identified the individual who committed the unsafe act. Virtually all such acts have a causal history that extends back in time and up through the levels of the system, however, and are most often attributable to latent conditions.

Latent Conditions
Latent conditions are the inevitable "resident pathogens," or flaws, within the work system.[40] They are present in all organizations. They stem from fallible decisions made by managers and top-level administrators, which give rise to poorly designed facilities, training gaps, staff shortages, heavy workload, and inadequate communication processes, policies, and procedures. Reason describes managers and top-level administrators at the "blunt end" of occurrences because they are removed in both space and time from the front line of direct, hands-on care delivery. Their influence is more indirect.

Latent conditions create two kinds of weaknesses in system defenses. One such weakness is longstanding unworkable procedures or design deficiencies in nursing work areas. As an example, the phone that nurses use to communicate with physicians is usually in the noisiest part of the care unit. Latent conditions can also create error-provoking conditions within the workplace that may lead to unsafe acts. Error-provoking conditions are characterized by time pressures, heavy workload, understaffing, high cognitive demands, interruptions, long hours, inadequate training, and unavailability of essential information.[40,41] Error-provoking conditions may overburden human limitations, causing active failure in nurses and an ultimate harmful event. Latent conditions, as the term suggests, may lie dormant for many years before they combine with active failures and local conditions to create an accident trajectory, as illustrated in Figure 12.2.

In the diagram, the accident sequence is from left to right.[27]

- The accident sequence begins with external environment pressures.
- Organizational management responds to the pressures and continues the sequence through the negative consequences of its decisions. An example is use of overtime to cope with a nursing shortage.
- The decisions are transmitted along departmental pathways to the work environment, where they create error-provoking conditions for unsafe acts. The error-provoking conditions overtax human abilities to perform the nursing activities adequately.
- The individual nurse commits an unsafe act, such as an attention slip, memory lapse, mistake during execution or decision making, or purposeful violation.
- A harmful event occurs.

Central to Reason's accident causation model is that the mental antecedents of unsafe acts are, beyond a certain point, extremely difficult to control.[27] Mental antecedents are what goes on in the mind of the health-care provider prior to the unsafe act. For example, the mental antecedents of distraction, momentary inattention, forgetting, losing the picture, preoccupation, and fixation are entirely natural human behaviors within an environment that can be hectic, demanding, time-pressured, and inadequately staffed. Unlike active failures, whose specific forms are often hard to foresee, latent conditions can be identified and remedied before harmful events occur.

Targeting latent conditions is a proactive strategy to prevent harmful events and is analogous to "health promotion" within the health-care system. Targeting latent conditions is more than simply treating the "illnesses" of health care by dealing with errors and harmful events as they occur; it involves determining and resolving the underlying cause for the patient care error and harmful event. The issue must be addressed from a broader perspective, with interventions directed toward changing the conditions in the health-care system that contribute to human error.

Nurses who have the greatest frequency of patient contact are uniquely positioned to detect and correct health-care errors before they reach the patient. Nurses are often the last line of defense against health-care errors.[42]

Although nurses are the safety nets, they are also the most vulnerable front-line care provider. Nurses inherit the latent conditions created by everyone else who has played a role in the inadequate design of the health-care delivery system. Rather than being the main instigators of an error leading to patient harm, nurses tend to be inheritors of system defects. "Their part is usually that of adding a final garnish to a lethal brew whose ingredients have already been long in the cooking."[40] Nurses and other health-care providers must be aware of the high-risk environment in which they work. A vital safety behavior in nurses is assertiveness in speaking up about latent conditions that put them and their patients at risk.

LATENT CONDITIONS IN THE NURSING WORK SYSTEM

These conditions, which affect nurse performance, include more acutely ill patients, shorter hospital stays, frequent patient turnover, extended hours and overtime, stressful work environments, interruption-driven environments, and high nursing workloads.

More Acutely Ill Patients

The increase in severity of illness of hospitalized patients requires a more sophisticated knowledge base to provide complex care treatments and a higher level of patient monitoring.[3]

Shorter Hospital Stays

Evidence is clear that sicker patients are staying in the hospital for shorter periods than in the past.[3] Reduced lengths of stay allow less time for nurses to become acquainted with their patients' baseline health or to develop the mental model and knowledge base required for critical thinking and decision making. There is less time for nurses to monitor, coordinate, and maintain continuity of care.[3]

Frequent Patient Turnover

A hospital bed may be occupied by more than one patient in a 24-hour period.[3] Patient turnover has been reported as high as 40% to 50% during an 8- to 12-hour period in some patient care units.[43] High patient turnover rates contribute to rapid admission-discharge cycles and increased workload for nurses. Assessing and stabilizing patients on admission, developing baseline knowledge, performing nursing safety activities, communicating with other health-care providers, providing patient education, and planning upon discharge are all time-condensed.[3] Time pressures increase cognitive and labor-intensive activities for nursing.

Extended Hours and Overtime

Nursing is hard work. It tires the mind, the body, and the emotions.[44] The use of extended work shifts and overtime has escalated as hospitals cope with the shortage of nurses. This latent condition, coupled with high patient acuity levels and rapid admission and discharge cycles, poses serious risks for the delivery of safe and effective care.[45] Prolonged work hours and fatigue have been demonstrated to cause lowered human performance and increased risk of error.[45,46] The effects of fatigue on human performance include a decline in reaction time, lapse of attention to detail, decreased concentration, working memory loss, slowing of thought processing, and decline in problem solving and decision making.[47]

Nursing associations have issued position statements regarding patient safety and nurse fatigue.[48,49] The position statements articulate the ethical responsibility registered nurses have to consider their level of fatigue when deciding whether to accept any assignment extending beyond the regularly scheduled work day or week, including a mandatory or voluntary overtime assignment. Clearly, large-scale system solutions are needed as both the United States and Canada face continued nursing shortages.

Stressful Work Environment

As stress increases, an individual's thought processes and breadth of attention narrow.[50-52] Stress increases the nurses' predisposition to human error. Essential to patient safety is the health-care professionals' ability to recognize the effects of stress on their human performance. Researchers have measured nurses' attitudes about stress. The results showed that 70% of all respondents believed that their decision-making abilities were as good in medical emergencies as in routine situations,[50] demonstrating that these nurses are in denial of the impact of stress and that susceptibility to error from stress is not acknowledged by health professionals. Health-care providers must become knowledgeable about the damaging effects of stress and the high risk for error that occurs in stressful situations.

Interruption-Driven Environment

Nurses and other health-care providers function within an interruption-driven work environment. Interruptions are latent system factors that have a marked effect on human performance, causing diversion of attention, stress, fatigue, forgetfulness, and error.[53-55] Interruptions are defined as an "uncontrollable and unpredictable stressor that results in information [overload] and cognitive fatigue. When interruptions cause an employee to leave tasks unfinished, these tasks act as distracters and further effort is required to inhibit attention to them while processing new inputs."[56]

A high frequency of interruptions can overburden a nurses' working memory. This may cause nurses to forget to do something important, such as calling a physician about an abnormal blood result, which may result in delays in treatment and increase the potential for patient harm.

Of great concern is that the nurse, whose attention is constantly shifting from one item to another during interruptions, may lose previously held information in working memory. Therefore, the nurse may not be able to formulate a complete and coherent clinical picture of the current state of her patients' needs.[20] Without a coherent clinical picture of the patient, critical thinking and clinical decision making will be affected. The potential for error is increased in an interruption-driven workplace. This in turn affects the accuracy of the patient clinical picture that is shared with other care providers.

Clearly, some interruptions are necessary to call attention to urgent situations; however, there is greater risk for human error when interruptions are the norm for communication. Safer work environments can be achieved through education, raising awareness of the consequences of interruptions on human abilities and patient safety, and the development of new strategies and technologies that minimize the need to generate interruptions in the first place.[55]

High Nursing Workload

Within an environment of numerous distractions and interruptions, nurses make clinical judgments about their patients, whose conditions are complex and may change minute by minute. A study conducted by Potter and colleagues[57] on the working conditions of nurses in acute care units revealed important information about the relationship among nurses' work, the work environment, and communication failures. During the course of work, nurses shift their focus and attention as they provide care from one patient to the next, an activity the researchers referred to as "cognitive shift." Nurses had an average of 76.6 cognitive shifts for their 12-hour shift, or 9.3 cognitive shifts per hour. Cognitive shifts demonstrate the challenge a nurse has in remembering the priorities and activities planned for a group of patients. Maintaining focus on the priorities and needs of multiple patients requires a sharp working memory. Researchers also calculated the nurses' cognitive stacking load, defined as everything the nurse needed to complete in the care of assigned patients at any given moment. Nurses' cognitive stacking load ranged from 11 to 21 activities. The study found that nurses were interrupted an average of 30 times during their shift. At the time nurses experienced an interruption, they had on average a cognitive stacking load of 15 activities. "Conceivably, a high cognitive stacking load may override the nurse's ability to properly attend to a given patient's priorities. Similarly, a high stacking load may lead to errors or omissions, particularly when further complicated by a high frequency of cognitive shifts and interruptions."[57]

Patient information in the nurses' working memory must remain active, particularly when new information from interruption competes for attention. Although harmful events did not occur, the nurses averaged four omissions during their shift. Omissions included missed assessments, incomplete patient education, missed interventions, and failure to communicate essential patient information to a health-care colleague.

CHAPTER SUMMARY

Communication failures among health-care team members are recognized as leading safety hazards. Nurses have the greatest amount of patient contact, and they communicate with other health-care providers as they continually monitor patient health status, coordinate and implement patient care services, and maintain continuity of care during transfers from one provider to another or one setting to another.

Nurses must be aware of the systems approach to managing errors in health-care settings. A systems approach views errors as the result of the consequences of organization system factors and emphasizes the importance of discovering how the system failed rather than focusing on the person making the error. This chapter presents an analysis of the nursing work system from a human factors science perspective. Within the nursing work system, the interactions between individual nurses, the nature of nursing work, the work environment, organizational management, and the external environment must support human performance abilities to produce optimal patient outcomes and quality care. Nurses must understand the nursing work system and how the work system design affects patient safety. Armed with this knowledge, nurses are able to anticipate and recognize mental antecedents of error within individuals and environmental conditions within systems, both of which result in patient harm.

BUILDING HIGH LEVEL COMMUNICATION COMPETENCE

For an interactive version of this activity, see DavisPlus at http://davisplus. fadavis.com

1. **Reflection:** Think about your initial reaction when you first read about the thousands of people who die every year in hospitals as a result of medical error. Have your thoughts changed about blaming individuals for errors?

2. Look up the words "sentinel" event and "adverse" event in the Patient-Safety Dictionary, located at http://rcpsc.medical.org/publications/patientsafety dictionary_e.pdf Watch the DVD on "Delivering Patient-safety" located on the homepage of the Canadian Patient-Safety Institute, located at www. patientsafetyinstitute.ca The video is approximately 9 minutes. Describe examples of communications between members of the health-care team to ensure the delivery of safe patient care.

References

1. Landrigan, C.P. The Handoff: A Critical Point of Vulnerability. CRICO/RM Forum March:6-7, 2007.
2. McCloskey, J., Bulechek, G. (eds.). Nursing Interventions Classification (NIC), 3rd ed. St Louis, Mosby: 2000.
3. Institute of Medicine. Page, A. (ed.). Keeping Patients Safe: Transforming the Work Environment of Nurses. Washington, D.C., National Academies Press: 2004.
4. Joint Commission on Accreditation of Healthcare Organizations. The Joint Commission Guide to Improving Staff Communication. Oakbrook Terrace, Ill., Joint Commissions Resources: 2005.
5. Clancy, C.M. Care Transitions: A Threat and an Opportunity for Patient Safety. American Journal of Medical Quality 1:415-417, 2006.
6. Hughes, R.G., Clancy, C.M. Improving the Complex Nature of Care Transitions. Journal of Nursing Care Quality 22:289-292, 2007.
7. Joint Commission. FAQs for the 2008 National Patient Safety Goals. Located at http://www.jointcommission.org/NR/rdonlyres/13234515-DD9A-4635-A718-D5E84A98AF13/0/2008_FAQs_NPSG_02.pdf Accessed January 2009.

8. Institute of Medicine. To Err Is Human: Building a Safer Health System: A Report of the Committee on Quality of Health Care in America. Washington, D.C., National Academies Press: 1999. Located at http://www.iom.edu/Object.File/Master/4/117/ToErr-8pager.pdf Accessed December 2008.
9. Leonard, M., Graham, S., Bonacum, D. The Human Factor: The Critical Importance of Effective Teamwork and Communication in Providing Safe Care. Quality and Safety in Health Care 13(S1):85-90, 2004.
10. Kohn, L.T., Corrigan, J.M., Donaldson, M.S. (eds.). To Err Is Human: Building a Safer Health System. Washington, D.C., National Academies Press, Institute of Medicine: 2000.
11. Frank, J.R., Brien, S. (eds.). The Safety Competencies: Enhancing Patient Safety Across the Health Professions. Ottawa, Ontario, Canada, Canadian Patient Safety Institute: 2008. Located at http://www.patientsafetyinstitute.ca/uploadedFiles/Safety_Competencies_16Sep08.pdf Accessed November 2008.
12. Bloomkatz, A. Goodness of Fit. Association of Psychological Science 18, 2005. Located at http://www.psychologicalscience.org/observer/getArticle.cfm?id=1826 Accessed January 2009.
13. Chapanis, A., Garner, W., Morgan, C. Applied Experimental Psychology: Human Factors in Engineering Design. N.Y., Wiley: 1985.
14. Henriksen, K., Dayton, E., Keyes, M.A., et al. Understanding Adverse Events: A Human Factors Framework. In Hughes, R.G. (ed.). Patient Safety and Quality: An Evidence-Based Handbook for Nurses. Rockville, Md., Agency for Healthcare Research and Quality: 2008.
15. Shappell, S.A., Wiegmann, D.A. The Human Factors Analysis and Classification System-HFACS. Springfield, Va., U.S. Department of Transportation Federal Aviation Administration: 2000. Located at http://www.nifc.gov/safety/reports/humanfactors_class&anly.pdf Accessed December 2008.
16. Feyer, A.M., Williamson, A.M. Human Factors in Accident Modeling. In Stellman, J.M. (ed). Encyclopedia of Occupational Health and Safety, 4th ed. Geneva, International Labour Organisation: 1998.
17. Chopra, V., Bovill, J.G., Spierdijk, J., et al. Reported Significant Observations During Anaesthesia: A Prospective Analysis Over an 18-Month Period. British Journal of Anaesthesia 68:13-17, 1992.
18. Cooper, J.B., Newbower, R.S., Long, C.D., et al. Preventable Anesthesia Mishaps: A Study of Human Factors. Quality and Safety in Health Care 11:277-282, 2002.
19. Donaldson, M.S. An Overview of To Err is Human: Re-emphasizing the Message of Patient Safety. In Hughes, R.G. (ed.). Patient Safety and Quality: An Evidence-Based Handbook for Nurses. Rockville, Md., Agency for Healthcare Research and Quality: 2008.
20. Cook, R.I., Woods, D.D. Operating at the Sharp End: The Complexity of Human Error. In Bogner, M.S. (ed.). Human Errors in Medicine. Hillsdale, N.J., Erlbaum: 1994.
21. Reason, J. Human Error. N.Y., Cambridge University Press: 1990.
22. Leape, L.L. Error in Medicine. Journal of the American Medical Association 272:1851-1857, 1994.
23. Hollnagel, E. Cognitive Ergonomics: It's All in the Mind. Ergonomics 40:1170-1182, 1997.
24. Parliamentary Office of Science and Technology. Managing Human Error. Postnote; June:1-8, 2001. Located at http://www.parliament.uk/post/pn156.pdf Accessed December 2008.
25. Reason, J. Managing the Risks of Organizational Accidents. Burlington, Vt., Ashgate: 1997.
26. Reason, J. Understanding Adverse Events: Human Events. Quality and Safety in Health Care 4:80-89, 1995.
27. Reason, J. Safety in the Operating Theatre: Human Error and Organizational Failure. Quality and Safety in Health Care 14:56-60, 2005.
28. Bacon, F. In Anderson, F. (ed.). The New Organon. Indianapolis, Bobbs-Merrill: 1960.
29. Koczmara, C., Jelincic, V., Dueck, C. 2005. Dangerous Abbreviations: "U" Can Make a Difference! CACCN 16:3, 12-15, 2005. Located at http://www.ismp-canada.org/download/CACCN-Fall05.pdf Accessed July 2008.
30. Tucker, A., Edmondson, A. Why Hospitals Don't Learn From Failures: Organizational and Psychological Dynamics That Inhibit System Change. California Management Review 45:55-72, 2003.
31. ElBardissi, A.W., Wiegmann, D.A., Dearani, J.A., et al. Application of the Human Factors Analysis and Classification System Methodology to the Cardiovascular Surgery Operating Room. Annals of Thoracic Surgery 83:1412-1419, 2007.
32. Vaughan, D. The Challenger Launch Decision: Risky Technology, Culture, and Deviance at NASA. Chicago, Chicago University Press: 1996.
33. Karsh, B-T., Alper, S.J. 2005. Work Systems Analysis: The Key to Understanding Health Care Systems. Rockville, Md., Agency for Healthcare Research and Quality: 2005. Located at http://www.ahrq.gov/downloads/pub/advances/vol2/Karsh.pdf Accessed January 2009.
34. Carayon, P., Hundt, A.S., Karsh, B. et al. Work System Design for Patient Safety: The SEIPS Model. Quality and Safety in Health Care 15:50-58, 2006.
35. Karsh, B., Holden, R.J., Alper, S.J., et al. A Human Factors Engineering Paradigm to Support the Performance of the Health Care Professional. Quality and Safety in Health Care 15:59-65, 2006.
36. Rousseau, D.M., House, R.J. Meso Organizational Behavior: Avoiding Three Fundamental Biases. In Cooper, C.L., Rousseau, D.M. (eds.). Trends in Organizational Behavior, vol. 1. John Wiley & Sons: 1994.

37. Vicente, K.J. What Does It Take: A Case Study. Joint Commission Journal on Quality and Safety. 29:598-609, 2003.

38. Vincent, C., Taylor-Adams, S., Stanhope, N. Framework for Analyzing Risk and Safety in Clinical Medicine. BMJ 316:1154-1157, 1998.

39. Smith, M.J., Karsh, B., Carayon. P., et al. Controlling Occupational Safety and Health Hazards. In Quick, J.C., Tetrick, L.E. (eds.). Handbook of Occupational Health Psychology. Washington, D.C., American Psychological Association: 2003.

40. Reason, J. 2000. Human Error: Models and Management. BMJ; 320; 768-770.

41. Ebright, P., Patterson, E., Chalko, B., et al. Understanding the Complexity of Registered Nurse Work in Acute Care Settings. Journal of Nursing Administration 33:630-638, 2003.

42. Hennerman, E.A., Gawlinski, A. A "Near-Miss" Model for Describing the Nurse's Role in the Recovery of Medical Errors. Journal of Professional Nursing 20:196-201, 2004.

43. Norrish, B., Rundall, T. Hospital Restructuring and the Work of Registered Nurses. Milbank Quarterly 79:55, 2001.

44. American Nurses Association. Nurse Fatigue. Located at http://www.nursingworld.org/MainMenu-Categories/ThePracticeofProfessionalNursing/workplace/Workforce/NurseFatigue.aspx Accessed December 2008.

45. Rogers, A.D., Hwang, W.T., Scott, L.D., et al. The Working Hours of Hospital Staff Nurses and Patient Safety. Health Affairs 23:202-212, 2004.

46. Dawson, D. Reid, K. Fatigue, Alcohol and Performance Impairment. Nature 388:235, 1997.

47. Van-Griever, A., Meijman, T. The Impact of Abnormal Hours of Work on Various Modes of Information Processing: A Process Model on Human Costs of Performance. Ergonomics 30:1287-1299, 1987.

48. American Nurses Association. 2006 Position Statements: Assuring Patient Safety: Registered Nurses' Responsibility in All Roles and Settings to Guard Against Working When Fatigued. Located at http://www.safestaffingsaveslives.org/WhatisSafeStaffing/MaketheCase/Fatigue.aspx Accessed January 2009.

49. College of Registered Nurses of Manitoba. 2004. Duty to Care. Located at http://cms.tng-secure.com/file_download.php?fFile_id=173 Accessed January 2009.

50. Sexton, J.B., Thomas, E.J., Helmreich, R.L. Error, Stress, and Teamwork in Medicine and Aviation: Cross-Sectional Surveys. BMJ 320:745-749, 2000.

51. Combs, A., Taylor, C. The Effect of the Perception of Mild Degrees of Threat on Performance. Journal of Abnormal Social Psychology 47:420-424, 1952.

52. Easterbrook, J.A. The Effect of Emotion on Cue Visualization and the Organization of Behavior. Psychological Review 66:183-201, 1959.

53. Edwards, M.B., Gronlund, S.D. Task Interruption and Its Effects on Memory. Memory 6:665-687, 1998.

54. Reitman, J.S. Without Surreptitious Rehearsal, Information in Short-Tem Memory Decays. Journal of Verbal Learning and Verbal Behavior 13:365-377, 1974.

55. Alvarez, G., Coiera, E. Interdisciplinary Communication: An Uncharted Source of Medical Error? Journal of Critical Care 21:236-242, 2006.

56. Kirmeyer, S. Coping With Competing Demands: Interruption and the Type A Pattern. Journal of Applied Psychology 73:621-629, 1988.

57. Potter, P., Wolf, L., Boxerman, S., et al. An Analysis of Nurses' Cognitive Work: A New Perspective for Understanding Medical Errors. In Henrikson, K., Battles, JB., Marks, E.S., et al. (eds.). Advances in Patient Safety: From Research to Implementation, vol. 1. Rockville, Md., Agency for Healthcare Research and Quality: 2005.

Health-Care Team Collaborative Patient-Safe Communication Strategies

13

Upon completion of this chapter, you will be able to:

1. Compare and contrast high-risk health-care organizations with non–health-care high-risk industries that have attained the status of high-reliability organizations.
2. Describe characteristics of effective groups and essential characteristics of group dynamics that are needed to build team collaboration and a culture of patient safety.
3. Identify stages of group process as they relate to health-care teams.
4. Identify behaviors of team members and team leaders that require high-level communication competency to promote group collaborative processes.
5. Describe conflict resolution strategies between health-care team members.
6. Identify health-care team communication patient-safe strategies designed to build safety into health care and prevent patient care errors.

Key Terms

Group process
SBAR
High-reliability organizations
Culture of safety
Handoff
Medication reconciliation
Tall man lettering
Readback/Hearback
Do Not Use list

Single-digit form
Concept Map Care Plan
Brief
Huddle
Debrief
DESC
CUS
Two-challenge rule

This chapter is focused on patient-safe strategies used by health-care team members as they work in groups to promote group collaboration to attain positive transformational outcomes within a culture of patient safety. The strategies promoting high-level communication processes to maintain collaborative working relationships for coordination of activities include brief, huddle, debrief, two-challenge rule, CUS, and DESC. Other patient-safe strategies discussed are those aimed at specific error-prone, high-risk communication situations that are well known to have led to patient harmful events in the health-care industry: patient handoff, readback/hearback, SBAR, Do Not Use list, medication reconciliation, single-digit form, and tall man lettering. Locate these strategies in the patient-safe strategies ring of the transformational model in Chapter 2. These strategies have been adapted from non–health-care high-risk industries.

High-risk industries that have sustained excellent records of success in maintaining safety and prevention of harmful events are called high-reliability organizations.[1] High-reliability non–health-care organizations are decades ahead of health-care organizations in building safety into their systems. Such organizations have learned from their own significant disasters, including those such as the *Challenger* launch decision,[2] airplane crashes,[3] the poison gas release at Bhopal, India,[4] and the nuclear reactor explosion at Chernobyl, Russia.[5] Major accidents like these affected the lives of many people. In comparison, accidents in health care typically involve one patient at a time and seem less dramatic.[6] Rarely do patient harmful events reach the headlines and public attention. Without the same impetus to improve safety that has been experienced by other industries, health care is the most poorly managed of all the high-risk industries and very late in coming to recognize the importance of system factors that underlie harmful events.[7]

This chapter begins with a comparison of health-care and other high-risk industries in developing a culture of safety. This leads to discussions of health-care team group communication principles and related patient-safe communication to promote group collaboration and synchronization. This chapter concludes with specific high-risk error-prone situations and the required patient-safe communication strategies to avoid harm to patients.

🧩 ORGANIZATIONAL CULTURE OF SAFETY

An organizational culture of safety refers to a commitment to safety that permeates all levels of an organization, from frontline personnel to executive management.[8] Individuals are encouraged to acknowledge the high-risk, error-prone nature of the organization's activities and voice concerns of any threats in the system before they cause harm.[9]

In a culture of safety, individuals are encouraged to report intercepted errors, errors, and harmful events, each of which can be discussed in an atmosphere of trust and mutual respect without fear of retribution.[10] Each reported incident provides an opportunity for organizations to learn about error and to identify error-provoking conditions in the system. By learning about errors, organizations can determine what safety improvements can be built into the system to reduce hazards, enhance human performance, and prevent errors from happening.[6] A culture of safety analyzes why and how errors happen rather than focusing on finding the person who might have been responsible.[11]

A culture of safety also encompasses a "just culture."[12] A just culture recognizes that people are fallible and acknowledges that even the most competent professional will make mistakes. Above all, a just culture does not hold professionals accountable for system failings over which they have no control. Nevertheless, a just culture does not tolerate conscious disregard of clear risks to patients or gross misconduct.[12]

A significant challenge for health-care organizations adopting the systems approach is to part with the traditional personal approach to errors that blames, names, shames, and retrains individuals who commit errors. This tradition stems from the traditional beliefs that individuals control their own destiny and are capable of choosing between right and wrong and that "bad" people make errors.[13]

High standards of performance are desirable in nurses, physicians, and other health-care providers, but such standards can become a serious problem when they create an expectation of perfection. Because nurses and physicians regard perfection as a professional standard, they feel shame when they make an error,[14] which creates pressure to hide or cover up errors.[15] As a result, rather than professionals and organizations openly discussing and learning from errors and system failures, errors are unreported. Without a detailed analysis of incidents and near misses, organizations have no way of uncovering recurrent system failures.[16] Systems that rely on perfection in human performance will result in failure. As spoken by Sir Liam Donaldson, Chief Medical Officer of the United Kingdom at the launch of the World Alliance for Patient Safety, "To err is human, to cover up is unforgivable, and to fail to learn is inexcusable."[17]

Although the health-care industry is similar to high-risk industries, it functions under even greater complexity.[18] High-risk non–health care industries operate with technical-intensive systems in which people interact with computer-automated processes. In comparison, health care is a person-intensive system largely composed of processes conducted by groups of people, not by computers. Members of health-care teams function as specialized groups using group processes to deliver health care to patients who have different and often unpredictable responses to care.

The development of curriculum and instructional ancillary materials to improve collaborative group processes is essential in making health care safer for all patients. Patient safety experts agree that communication is essential for the provision of quality health care and the prevention and correction of human errors leading to patient injury and harm.[19] Currently, most health-care curricula lack teamwork principles and practices that are essential to achieving high reliability in health-care organization, even when evidence suggests that failures in teamwork and communication underlie most sentinel events.[19]

Standardized processes to create a shared model of patients' situations are essential. One type of model is the Concept Map Care plan.[20] Currently used in nursing education, the concept care map is developed from a multidisciplinary perspective and allows team members to visualize the interrelationships between medical diagnoses, nursing diagnoses, assessment data, and treatments. This holistic perspective gives team members a clear picture of the patient's clinical situation, including the relationships between medical and nursing care problems, with integration of pathology, medications, treatments, and laboratory and diagnostic testing.[20] Errors are more likely to be detected before harm occurs.

In the health-care system, there are too few standards and safe practices focused on interdisciplinary patient-safe communication strategies. Communication variations go unchecked because expected behaviors have not been adequately established. Lack of adequate standards in patient-safe communication is the epidemic that plagues patient safety from a systems perspective. All too frequently, communication is situation- or personality-dependent and left open to chance. Accepted ambiguity in communication as a result of poorly defined communication expectations leads to inadvertent patient harm.[21]

Standards for Team Communication

First and foremost, all members of the health-care team must have excellent communication skills. Team members need to have the ability to actively listen and encourage others, to share in a team member's success or failure, and have the capability to know a colleague well.[22] Box 13.1 provides strategies used by individuals to promote effective communication and collaboration.

BOX 13.1 *Strategies for Effective Communication and Collaboration in Health Care Teams*[23]

- Be respectful and professional.
- Listen actively.
- Try to understand the other person's viewpoint.
- Model an attitude of collaboration, and expect it.
- Identify the bottom line. Decide what is negotiable and non-negotiable in patient care management; for example, patient safety is not negotiable; when staff members take a break is negotiable.
- Acknowledge the other person's thoughts and feelings.
- Pay attention to your own ideas and what you have to offer the group.
- Be cooperative.
- Be direct.
- Identify common, shared goals and concerns.
- State your feelings using "I" statements.
- Do not take things personally.
- Learn to say "I was wrong" and "You could be right."
- Do not feel pressure to agree instantly.
- Think about all possible solutions before a meeting, and be willing to adapt if a more creative alternative is presented.
- Recognize that negotiation and resolution of conflict takes time and may require several interactions.

All team members must understand group processes and the stages of small group development.[24-26] Group process refers to an understanding of the behavior of people in groups trying to solve problems and make decisions. Health-care providers must be able to apply knowledge of group processes to health-care team processes.

Stages of classic group process have been described in the classic work of Tuckman and Jensen[24,25] and include the stages of forming, storming, norming, performing, and adjourning, as shown in Box 13.2.

> **BOX 13.2** *Stages of Group Process Applied to Health-Care Teams*
>
> *Forming:* Relationship development: team orientation, identification of role expectations, beginning team interactions, explorations, and boundary setting.
> *Storming:* Interpersonal interaction and reaction: dealing with tension, conflict, and confrontation.
> *Norming:* Effective cooperation and collaboration: personal opinions are expressed and resolution of conflict with formation of solidified goals and increased group cohesiveness.
> *Performing:* Group maturity and stable relationships: team roles become more functional and flexible, structural issues are resolved leading to supportive task performance through group-directed collaboration and resource sharing.
> *Adjourning:* Termination and consolidation: team goals were met, closure occurs after evaluation, and review of outcomes.

Nursing students must also become aware how group member status and power affect communication processes of groups. Status is the measure of worth conferred on an individual by a group and profoundly affects group processes.[27]

Team Member Status

A report by the Institute of Medicine[28] on "Keeping Patients Safe: Transforming the Work Environment of Nurses" suggested that status differences affect patient outcomes and are partly responsible for many patient care errors. In a review of medical malpractice cases, Schmitt[29] suggested that physicians who were perceived by some as higher-status members often ignored important information communicated by nurses, who were perceived by some to be lower-status members of the team. Nurses in turn were found to withhold relevant information related to monitoring patients from physicians perceived as intimidating to them. It is important to develop a team where all members are trusted and respected for their roles in attaining the team's goals of high-quality care.

Nurses are educated in team leadership roles and must possess the knowledge to ensure that team members are sharing information, helping each other when needed, and resolving conflicts. The coordination of a team requires high-level communication competency. The specific patient-safe communication behaviors required of team leaders are shown in Box 13.3.

> **BOX 13.3** *Effective Team Leader Behaviors*[19]
>
> • Organizes the team: utilizes resources to maximize performance, balances workload, and delegates tasks and assignments as appropriate.
> • Articulates clear goals.
> • Makes decisions based on input of team members.
> • Empowers team members to speak up and openly challenge, when appropriate.
> • Promotes and facilitates good teamwork; e.g., briefs, huddles, debriefs.
> • Resolves conflict; e.g., uses the two-challenge rule, CUS, and DESC.

Promotion and facilitation of teamwork by the nursing team leader can be accomplished through the following patient-safe strategies that are standardized processes from high-reliability organizations and have been adapted to health-care teams to minimize patient care errors:

Brief
A brief is a short planning session prior to the start of team activities to discuss team formation, assign roles, establish expectations, and anticipate outcomes. Briefs clarify who will be leading the team so others know where to look for guidance, and open lines of communication to ensure that members can contribute their unique knowledge to the tasks to be accomplished. Protocols, responsibilities, and expected behaviors are discussed and reinforced so that misunderstandings are avoided and disruptive or unexpected behaviors are potentially avoided.

Huddle
A huddle is a problem-solving session to establish situation awareness so that all team members know updates in the current situation, are aware of what is going on around them, and share the same mental model. The team assesses the need to adjust the initial plans.

Debrief
The debrief is a means to improve group processes through an informal information session to review team performance after completion of activities. It addresses what went well and what should change or improve. There is a recap of the key events that occurred and lessons learned, and goals are set for improvement.

One of the most important functions of the group team leader is conflict resolution. The standard conflict resolution processes from high-reliability organizations are outlined as follows:

Resolving Conflict Through Feedback
Team members must advocate for the patient and assertively state corrective actions in a firm and respectful manner by stating the concern, offering a solution, and obtaining agreement. "I am concerned about the drop in your patient's blood pressure. How should we address this?" If this is ignored, use the two-challenge rule.

Two-Challenge Rule
Assertively voice your concern at least *two times* to ensure it was heard, and the team member being challenged must acknowledge the feedback. If you still believe patient or staff safety may be compromised after discussion with the team member, then take additional action by contacting a supervisor, and communicate the situation to the entire team. If you are challenged, you must acknowledge the concerns. Every team member needs to be empowered to stop safety breaches.

CUS
This is a technique to provide a framework for conflict resolution using signal words for patient safety. First state your *concern*, "I am concerned about [complete]." Then state why you are *uncomfortable*: "I am uncomfortable because [complete]." Then state why this is a *safety issue*: "This is a safety issue because [complete]."

DESC

A team leader uses DESC when a conflict becomes personal in nature and team members become hostile toward one another, affecting their performance and safe patient care. The team leader sits down with the conflicting parties, who *describe* the specific situation or behavior, providing concrete data; *express* how the situation makes them feel/what the concerns are; *suggest* other alternatives and seek agreement; and state the *consequences* of the behaviors in terms of impact on established team goals. The conflicting parties should strive for consensus. When using DESC, the team leader works on a win-win outcome despite the interpersonal conflict, stressing that team unity and quality of care are dependent on coming to an agreement all parties can accept.

In the last section of this book, we examine specific patient-safe communication strategies that facilitate effective communications between members of the health-care team that have been adopted from high-reliability organizations. These patient-safe strategies have been designed to overcome health-care system weaknesses that have resulted in patient care errors, and they support the national patient safety goal of improving communication among health-care providers in the United States and Canada.

HIGH-RELIABILITY PATIENT-SAFE COMMUNICATION STRATEGIES

Communication standardized processes in high-reliability organizations are termed "safety nets" because they describe behavior expected of individuals that ensures high-quality performance: health-care organizations have adopted standardized communication processes from high-reliability organizations to be used as patient-safe communication strategies including:

- Guidelines for effective handoff
- Medication reconciliation at transitions in care
- Guidelines for written documentation in health records
- Strategies to avoid errors due to look-alike/sound-alike medications
- Readback/hearback when accepting and transcribing verbal and telephone orders
- SBAR (Situation-Background-Assessment-Recommendation) tool when communicating changes or updates in patient condition

Handoff: A Critical Point of Vulnerability

A handoff is the transfer of essential patient information and responsibility of care from one care provider to another for the purpose of ensuring continuity in care and patient safety.[30] It is recognized as the highest point of vulnerability in patient safety.[31-33] Terms in nursing that are synonymous with handoff include report, nursing report, or shift report. Handoffs occur during the following transitions in care:

- Nurse-to-nurse
- Shift-to-shift
- Unit-to-unit
- Facility-to-facility

The handoff includes communication methods between the health-care providers such as verbal, written, or simultaneous verbal and written channels and is dependent on the health-care providers' communication competency, level of stress, fatigue, or overload. It is performed in a work environment with time pressures and interruptions and is influenced by existing communication norms and organizational culture.

The handoff is a complex process. It must provide accurate essential information, including the patient's current status, recent changes in condition or treatment, anticipated changes in condition or treatment to watch for, and plans that may be considered to address anticipated events.[34]

The handoff creates an accurate mental model of the patient situation, bringing attention to care that is in progress as well as contingency planning for the next interval of care. A nursing study demonstrated that simply listing historical events is not as effective in conveying mental models of the situation as is describing problems, hypotheses, and predictive assessment of the situation.[35] Communications between health-care providers during handoff allow the individual accepting responsibility for the patient to ask questions to clarify and verify the details and to confirm understanding so that differences in mental models can be exposed.[36]

The handoff provides opportunity for the individual who is accepting responsibility of the patient to bring a fresh perspective to the patient situation. A fresh perspective can detect fixation errors caused by fatigued decision making.[37,38] Recall from Chapter 12 that fixation means that a health-care provider sees only the information that confirms personal expectations rather than seeing the information that is actually present and that might contradict what is expected. Questions such as, "Do you know that for sure?" or "Did you try this?" detect fixation errors. Handoff is an integral communication process between health-care providers that promotes effective critical thinking and decision making, maintains continuity of care, and promotes patient safety.

The result of inadequate handoffs is that safety often fails,[39] resulting in, for example, wrong-site surgery,[40] medications errors,[41] mismanagement of critical results,[42] and patient deaths.[42,43]

Multiple and recurring handoffs in serial fashion may result in the potential for a progressive loss of information if certain information is missed, forgotten, or otherwise not conveyed.[44,45] "As a result, while the demand for accurate and timely information has increased, the likelihood that this same information is fragmented across care providers has also increased. This apparent paradox jeopardizes patient safety."[44]

In high-reliability organizations, standardized handoff procedures are practiced hundreds of times to ensure that no information is lost during the transfer of information.[46] But in health care, this is not the case. In one study, only 8% of medical schools taught students how to hand off patients in a formal process.[47] Nursing programs may include communication theory, but they do not teach the specific handoff process.[48] Instead, handoffs have been taught by preceptors, with medical and nursing students watching how they have given and received handoffs. Each preceptor may hand off differently, leaving students unsure of best practice.[45]

Despite being noted as the most vulnerable point in communication, there is surprisingly little in the literature that suggests characteristics of a "good" handoff and what form it should take (written, verbal, or both) to be most effective. Because nurses hand off information about patients so often, they may not realize handoff communication is a high-risk process.[49] Nurses have described high variability in the level of information given during change of shift handoff reports.[50,51] Handoff that occurs at the beginning of a shift has always been an important part of the communication process in nursing, providing focus and direction to nurses beginning their shift, and helping to maintain continuity of care.

The quality of handoff influences directly the delivery of care for the shift that follows.[52] Several studies demonstrate that the actual content of the information handed over is inconsistent, with insufficient and nonspecific detail. Information is often subjective and includes jargon, abbreviations, and poor descriptors, including "fine" or "OK." Often the only consistency is giving the patient's name, age, resuscitation status, diagnosis, and treatment, reflecting more of a medical model with little reference to nursing care.[53-55] Sherlock[54] found that the only time the verbal report was more detailed was when the patient's condition was critical rather than stable. The content of handoff lacked standardization, and the quality of the information was dependent on the person giving the report. As a result, essential care was not communicated consistently. These studies demonstrate the need for improvement, organization, and standardization in the quality of patient information presented at handoff.

Patterson[46] examined the handoff communication strategy used in high-reliability organizations including NASA, Canadian nuclear power plants, a U.S. railroad dispatch center, and an ambulance dispatch center in Toronto, Canada. The handoff characteristics that these high-reliability organizations all shared included:

- Face-to-face verbal update with interactive questioning
- Topics initiated by the person assuming responsibility as well as the person being replaced
- Repeating back by the incoming person to ensure information was accurately interpreted
- Information presented in the same order every time
- Limited interruptions
- Written summary of activities that occurred during the shift

Following the guidelines established by high-reliability organizations, the World Health Organization Collaborating Center and other leading organizations have developed health-care handoff recommendations. The guidelines reflect the communication process in the transformational model with focus on the creation of common meaning and also include creation of a shared mental model of the patient situation. The recommendations are as follows[47,56,57]:

- Use clear and common language; avoid jargon, ambiguous words, or confusing terms that are open to misinterpretation.
- Limit interruptions during handoff communications.
- Focus on the information being exchanged; avoid distractions, such as mixing a medication or trying to chart at the same time as listening to another's handoff.
- Allocate sufficient time for handoff.
- Encourage interactive questioning, allowing opportunity to verify and clarify information.
- At minimum, include diagnosis, allergies, current condition, recent changes in condition, ongoing treatment, and possible changes or complications that might occur and what the plan of action should be if complications do occur in the next time interval.

Medication Reconciliation at Handoff

A key consideration during handoff is the reliability of medication information. Medication regimes must be carefully communicated between health-care providers: 46%

of medication errors occur when new orders are written at patient admission and discharge.[58] The World Health Organization Collaborating Center has recommended a verification process of medication reconciliation to prevent medication errors at care transition points[59]:

* Write a complete and accurate list of all medications the patient is taking at home.
* Compare the list against the admission, transfer, and discharge orders, and bring discrepancies to the attention of the prescribing physician.
* Keep the list updated.
* Communicate the list to the next provider of care whenever the patient is transferred from one care unit to another and when the patient is discharged home.
* Keep the list in a visible location on the patient's chart.

Guidelines for Written Documentation in Health Records

In the health setting, the patient's chart contains the written documentation of assessments, treatments, and patient responses to interventions and medically prescribed therapies. The chart is a communication tool in which essential patient information is recorded and shared by all members of the interdisciplinary health-care team. From the shared pool of interdisciplinary information, clinical decisions are made, and continuity of care is maintained across care providers and nursing shifts. Therefore, it is imperative that documentation is interpreted as intended. Illegible handwriting and use of abbreviations and symbols create error-prone conditions in health care. Factors such as time pressures, noise, and interruptions can increase the likelihood of misinterpretations and human error.

The World Health Organization Collaborating Center[56] has recommended that health-care providers print drug names and dosages. The Joint Commission[57] and the Institutes for Safe Medication Practices in the United States[60] and Canada[61] have recommended elimination of the use of dangerous abbreviations, acronyms, and symbols in written communications. Guidelines for Do Not Use abbreviations and symbols have been developed by each organization. Health-care agencies can tailor the Do Not Use list specific to their independent analysis of incidents and harmful events.

Interpretation of abbreviations and symbols is vulnerable to confirmation bias. Confirmation bias, where health-care providers will see what they expect to see, is influenced by factors such as stress, fatigue, and time pressures. Confirmation bias can lead to errors in interpretation of the intended meaning of written physician orders, so keep these patient safe practices in mind:

* The letters U, u, and IU have been used as an abbreviation for the word "units"; *patient-safe practice:* instead of U, u, or IU, write units[60]
* Written Latin abbreviations, although the norm in medicine, can lead to misinterpretations; *patient-safe practice:* instead of QD, write daily; instead of QOD, write every other day[60]
* Always use a zero before a decimal point for a fractionated dosage: e.g., 0.5 mg[60]
* Tenfold dosage errors can also occur with trailing zeros; *patient-safe practice:* do not write a zero after a decimal point, and do not use a decimal point for a non-fractionated drug dosage; write, for example, 1 mg[60]

Strategies to Avoid Errors Due to Look-Alike/Sound-Alike Medications

With tens of thousands of medications available, over 600 pairs of look-alike and sound-alike drug names have been reported.[62] The potential for error is significant. In terms of look-alike drugs, contributing to risk of misinterpretation are illegible handwriting, the care providers' unfamiliarity with drug names, new products, similar packaging, similar clinical uses, and the failure of pharmaceutical manufacturers to recognize potential for error prior to approving new drug names.[63,64] The World Health Organization Collaborating Center has recommended that drug name differences should be emphasized using methods such as "tall man" lettering. Examples of tall man lettering are LamiCTAL and LamiSIL.[65]

Readback/Hearback: Accepting and Transcribing Verbal and Telephone Orders

Nurses receive face-to-face and phone orders from physicians and advanced nurse practitioners for patient medications and treatments on a daily basis. They receive critical results over the phone from the laboratory and other information from radiology and the many disciplines involved in the patient's care. The transfer of patient information verbally and over the phone translates into clinical decision-making and nursing actions; therefore, accuracy in communications is vital to ensure patient safety. A patient-safe communication strategy for accepting and transcribing face-to-face and phone orders with accuracy is readback/hearback.[66] It is an essential ground rule for communication among members of groups managing complex, high-consequence processes, such as aviation and other high-reliability organizations.[67] Ensuring that messages are clearly received and understood as intended requires "readback/hearback" described in the following sequence[66]:

- The sender states information concisely to the receiver.
- The receiver writes the information down *first* and reads back what has been written.
- The sender provides a hearback acknowledging that the readback was correct or makes a correction.
- The readback/hearback process continues until a shared understanding is mutually verified.

Readback/hearback efficiently guides communication among two or more people to a verified mutual understanding, helping them to avoid errors arising from informational gaps and miscommunications.[66] *Only the individual giving the verbal order can verify it as accurate against what was intended.*[68]

Situation-Background-Assessment-Recommendation

NASA and commercial aviation have shown that the adoption of standardized communication tools and behaviors is a very effective strategy in reducing risk of harmful events.[46] This is particularly true when there is a power or authority gradient between two communicators. For example, in health care, a physician is considered at the top of the hierarchy and has more authority than a nurse. Physicians often do not receive critical information because nurses may be unable to speak in a clear and assertive way and overcome the authority gradient. One such tool that standardizes behavior between physicians and nurse is the situation, background, assessment, and recommendation (SBAR) instrument. The SBAR tool for communication includes[21,69]:

S—Situation. Describe the problem in a simple sentence. What is going on with the patient?

B—Background. What is the clinical background or context? Anticipate the listener's questions about the situation, and provide the answers.

A—Assessment. Summarize your observations about the situation. What do you think the problem is?

R—Recommendation. Provide a specific recommendation for problem solving.

The use of such a tool forces both the sender and receiver to move through a discussion in a predictable, logical flow that is not dependent on personality, status or hierarchy, sex, ethnic background,[70] or differences in communication styles between nurses and physicians.[71] It allows health-care providers with differing communication styles to speak the same language. It does not leave communication open to chance.

Briefly and concisely, critically important pieces of information have been transmitted in a predictable structure. Not only is there familiarity in how health-care providers communicate, but the SBAR develops critical thinking skills as the person initiating the conversation knows to indicate the problem, provide an assessment, and indicate appropriate treatments.[21]

CHAPTER SUMMARY

High-risk industries have high potential for errors with disastrous consequences. Health-care organizations are high-risk industries that have lagged behind other high-risk industries in adopting a systems approach because health-care errors have not received the same attention as public disasters that have occurred in other industries. Since 2000, when the initial Institute of Medicine report on errors in health care was published, and health-care providers became fully aware of the magnitude of patient-care errors, there has been an impetus in health-care organizations to promote a culture of patient safety and build a safer health-care system.

A culture of patient safety and building safety into a health-care system depends on communication that facilitates collaboration between members of the health-care team. Communication failures are the leading safety hazard in health care and result in a lack of collaboration between members of the interdisciplinary health-care team.

BUILDING HIGH-LEVEL COMMUNICATION COMPETENCE

For additional exercises, see DavisPlus at http://davisplus.fadavis.com

1. **Reflection.** Think about the team leaders with whom you have worked during your clinical rotations. What skills do they exhibit? How do they exhibit them?

2. **Practice.** Work with a colleague, and practice readback/hearback and the SBAR.

3. **Critical Thinking.** How do communication standards and structured communications improve patient safety?

References

1. Weick, K., Sutcliffe, K. Managing the Unexpected: Assuring High Performance in an Age of Complexity. San Francisco, Jossey-Bass: 2001.
2. Vaughan, D. The *Challenger* Launch Decision: Risky Technology, Culture, and Deviance at NASA. Chicago, Chicago University Press: 1996.
3. MacPherson, M. The Black Box: Cockpit Voice Recorder Accounts of In-Flight Accidents. London, Harper Collins: 1998.
4. Perrow, C. Normal Accidents: Living With High-Risk Technologies. New Jersey, Princeton University Press: 1999.
5. Reason, J. Managing the Risks of Organizational Accidents. Burlington, Vt., Ashgate Publishing: 1997.
6. Institute of Medicine. Kohn, L.T., Corrigan, J.M., Donaldson, M.S. (eds.). To Err Is Human: Building a Safer Health System. Washington, D.C., National Academy Press: 2000.
7. Henriksen, K., Dayton, E., Keyes, M.A., et al. Understanding Adverse Events: A Human Factors Framework. In Hughes, R.G. (ed.). Patient Safety and Quality: An Evidence-Based Handbook for Nurses. Rockville, Md., AHRQ Publication No. 08-0043: 2008.
8. Weick, K.E. 1987. Organizational Culture as a Source of High Reliability. California Management Review 29:112-127, 1987.
9. Pizzi, L., Goldfarb, N., Nash, D. Promoting a Culture of Safety. In Shojania, K.G., Duncan, B.W., McDonald, K.M., et al. (eds.). Making Health Care Safer: A Critical Analysis of Patient Safety Practices. Rockville, Md., AHRQ Publication No. 01-E058: 2001.
10. Farquhar, M., Collins Sharp, B.A., Clancy, C.M. Patient Safety in Nursing Practice. Association of Perioperative Registered Nurses Journal 86: 455-457, 2007.
11. Hughes, R.G. First, Do No Harm: Avoiding the Near Misses. American Journal of Nursing 104:81-84, 2004.
12. Marx, D. Patient Safety and the "Just Culture": A Primer for Health Care Executives. New York, Columbia University: 2001. Available at: http://www.mers-tm.org/support/Marx_Primer.pdf
13. Langer, E.J. The Psychology of Control. Beverly Hills, Sage: 1983.
14. Leape, L.L. Error in Medicine. Journal of the American Medical Association 272:1851-1857, 1994.
15. Wakefield, D., Wakefield, B., Uden-Holman, T., et al. Perceived Barriers in Reporting Medication Administration Errors. Best Practices and Benchmarking in Healthcare 1:191-197, 1996.
16. Reason, J. Human Error: Models and Management. British Medical Journal 320:768-770, 2000.
17. Donaldson, L. Building the Safest Health System 2008-2013: Strategic Plan. Washington, D.C., Canadian Patient Safety Institute: 2008.
18. Ternov, S. The Human Side of Medical Mistakes. In Spath, P.L. (ed.). Error Reduction in Heath Care: A Systems Approach to Improving Patient Safety. Jossey-Bass:1999.
19. Agency for Healthcare Research and Quality. Instructor Guide for TeamSTEPPS: Team Strategies & Tools to Enhance Performance and Patient Safety. Rockville, Md., AHRQ Pub. No. 06-0020: 2006.
20. Schuster, P. Concept Mapping: A Critical Thinking Approach to Care Planning, 2nd ed. Philadelphia, FA Davis: 2008.
21. Joint Commission. Sentinel Event Statistics, June 29, 2004. In Leonard, M., Graham, S., Bonacum, D. (eds.). The Human Factor: The Critical Importance of Effective Teamwork and Communication in Providing Safe Care. Quality and Safety in Health Care. 13:i85-i90, 2004.
22. Dziabis, S.P., Lant T.W. Building Partnerships With Physicians: Moving Outside the Walls of the Hospital. Nursing Administration Quarterly 22:1-5, 1998.
23. Rider, E. Twelve Strategies for Effective Communication and Collaboration in Medical Teams. British Medical Journal 325:S45, 2002.
24. Tuckman, B.W. Developmental Sequences in Small Groups. Psychological Bulletin 63:384-399, 1965.
25. Tuckman, B. W., Jensen, M.A.C. Stages of Small Group Development Revisited. Group and Organizational Studies 2:419-427, 1977.
26. O'Daniel, M., Rosenstein, A.H. Professional Communication and Team Collaboration. In Hughes, R.G. (ed.). Patient Safety and Quality: An Evidence-Based Handbook for Nurses. Rockville, Md., Agency for Healthcare Research and Quality: 2008.
27. Scott, W.G. Organizational Theory. Homewood, Ill.: Irwin, 1967.
28. Page, A. (ed.). Keeping Patients Safe: Transforming the Work Environment of Nurses. Washington, D.C., National Academies Press: 2004.
29. Schmitt, M.H. Collaboration Improves the Quality of Care: Methodological Challenges and Evidence From U.S. Health Care Research. Journal of Interprofessional Care, 15:47-66, 2001.
30. National Quality Forum. Safe Practices for Better Health Care 2006 Update. Washington, D.C, 2007.
31. Australian Council for Safety and Quality in Health Care 2005. Clinical Handover and Patient Safety Literature Review Report. Available at http://www..safetyandquality.org/index.cfm?page=Publications# clinhovrlit Accessed December 2008.

32. Donchin, Y., Gopher, D., Olin, M., et al. A Look Into the Nature and Causes of Human Errors in the Intensive Care Unit. Quality and Safety in Health Care 12:143-147, 2003.
33. Cooper, J.B., Newbower, R.S., Long, C.D., et al. Preventable Anesthesia Mishaps: A Study of Human Factors. Quality and Safety in Health Care 11:277-282, 2002.
34. Joint Commission. FAQs for the 2008 National Patient Safety Goals. Located at http://www.jointcommission. org/NR/rdonlyres/13234515-DD9A-4635-A718-D5E84A98AF13/0/2008_FAQs_NPSG_02.pdf Accessed January 2009.
35. Kihlgrhen, M., Lindsten, I., Norberg, A., et al. The Content of the Oral Daily Reports at a Long-Term Care Ward Before and After Staff Training in Integrity-Promoting Care. Scandinavian Journal of Caring Science 6:105-112, 1992.
36. Grusenmeyer, C. Shared Functional Representation in Cooperative Tasks: The Example of Shift Changeover. International Journal of Human Factors in Manufacturing 5:163-179, 1995.
37. DeKeyser, V., Woods, D.D. Fixation Errors: Failures to Revise Situation Assessment in Dynamic and Risky Systems. In Columbo, A.G., Saiz de Bustamante, A. (eds.). Systems Reliability Assessment. Amsterdam, Kluwer: 1990.
38. Lardner, R. Effective Shift Handover: A Literature Review. Offshore Technology Report, 1996. Located at http://www.hse.gov.uk/research/otopdf/1996/oto96003.pdf
39. Institute of Medicine. Crossing the Quality Chasm: A New Health System for the 21st Century. Washington, D.C., National Academies Press: 2001.
40. Sanchez, R.R. When a Medical Mistake Becomes a Media Event: Interview by Mark Crane. Journal of Medical Economics 74:158-162, 165-168, 170-171, 1997.
41. Hicks, R.W., Santell, J.P., Cousins, D.D., et al. MEDMARX 5th Anniversary Data Report: A Chartbook of 2003 Findings and Trends 1999-2003. Rockville, Md., USP Center for Advancement of Patient Safety: 2004.
42. Gandhi, T.K. Fumbled Handoffs: One Dropped Ball After Another. Annals of Internal Medicine 142:352-358, 2005.
43. Beach, C. Morbidity & Mortality Rounds: Lost in Transition. Located at http://webmm.ahrq.gov/case.aspx?caseID=116
44. Anthony, M.K., Preuss, G. Models of Care: The Influence of Nurse Communication on Patient Safety. Located at http://findarticles.com/p/articles/mi_m0FSW/is_5_20/ai_n18614298 Accessed January 2009.
45. Dracup, K., Morris, P.E. Passing the Torch: The Challenge of Handoffs. American Journal of Critical Care. 17:95-97, 2008.
46. Patterson, E.S., Roth, E.M., Woods, D.D., et al. Strategies in Settings With High Consequences for Failure: Lessons for Health Care Operations. International Journal for Quality in Health Care 16:125-132, 2004.
47. Solet, D.J., Norvell, J.M., Rutan G.H., et al. Lost in Translation: Challenges and Opportunities in Physician-to-Physician Communication During Patient Handoffs. Academic Medicine 80:1094-1099, 2005.
48. Friesen, M.A., White, S.V., Byers, J.F. Handoffs: Implications for Nurses. In Hughes R.G. (ed.). Patient Safety and Quality: An Evidence-Based Handbook for Nurses. Rockville, Md., Agency for Healthcare Research and Quality: 2008.
49. Porto, G. Focus on Five: Strategies to Improve Handoff Communication—Implementing a Process to Resolve Questions. Joint Commission Perspectives on Patient Safety 5, 2005.
50. Clancy, C.M. Care Transitions: A Threat and an Opportunity for Patient Safety. American Journal of Medical Quality 1:415-417, 2006.
51. Hughes, R.G., Clancy, C.M. Improving the Complex Nature of Care Transitions. Journal of Nursing Care Quality 22:289-292, 2007.
52. Thurgood, G. Verbal Handover Reports: What Skills Are Needed? British Journal of Nursing 4:720-722, 1995.
53. Parker, J., Gardner, G., Wiltshire, J. Handover: The Collective Narrative of Nursing Practice. Australia Journal of Advanced Nursing 9:31-37, 1992.
54. Sherlock, C. The Patient Handover: A Study of Its Form, Function, and Efficiency. Nursing Standard 52:33-36, 1995.
55. Payne, S. Interactions Between Nurses During Handovers in Elderly Care. Journal of Advanced Nursing 32:275-277, 2000.
56. World Health Organization. Communication During Patient Handovers: Patient Safety Solutions. 1, 2007.
57. Joint Commission. Focus on Five: Strategies to Improve Handoff Communication—Implementing a Process to Resolve Questions. Joint Commission Perspectives on Patient Safety 5, 2005.
58. Forster, A.J., Clark, H.D., Menard, A., et al. Adverse Events Among Medical Patients After Discharge From Hospital. Canadian Medical Association Journal 170(3):345-349, 2004.
59. World Health Organization. Assuring Medication Accuracy at Transitions in Care. Patient Safety Solutions 1, 2007.

60. Institute for Safe Medication Practices. ISMP's List of Error-Prone Abbreviations, Symbols and Dose Designations. Located at http://www.ismp.org/Tools/errorproneabbreviations.pdf
61. Institute for Safe Medication Practices Canada. Eliminate Use of Dangerous Abbreviations, Symbols, and Dose Designations. Located at http://www.ismp-canada.org/download/safetyBulletins/ISMPCSB2006-04Abbr.pdf
62. Institute for Safe Medication Practices. Please Don't Sleep Through This Wake Up Call. ISMP Medication Safety Alert 6:1, 2001.
63. McCoy, LK. Look-Alike, Sound-Alike Drugs Review: Include Look-Alike Packaging as an Additional Safety Check. Joint Commission Journal on Quality and Patient Safety 31:47-53, 2005.
64. Hoffman, J.M., Proulx, S.M. Medication Errors Caused by Drug Name Confusion. Drug Safety 26:445-452, 2003.
65. World Health Organization. Look-Alike, Sound-Alike Medication Names. Patient Safety Solutions 1, 2007.
66. Brown, J.P. Closing the Communication Loop: Using Readback/Hearback to Support Patient Safety. Joint Commission Journal on Quality and Safety 30:460-464, 2004.
67. Aeronautical Information Manual: Official Guide to Basic Flight Information and Air Traffic Control. Section 2, Radio Communication Phraseology and Techniques. Washington, D.C., U.S. Department of Transportation, Federal Aviation Administration: 2008.
68. Cohen, M.R. Medication Errors: Causes, Prevention and Risk Management. Washington, D.C., American Pharmaceutical Association Foundation, 1999.
69. Haig, K.M., Sutton, S., Whittington, J. SBAR: A Shared Mental Model for Improving Communication Between Clinicians. Journal on Quality and Patient Safety 32:167-175, 2006.
70. Thomas, E.J., Sexton, J.B., Helmreich, R.L. Discrepant Attitudes About Teamwork Among Critical Care Nurses and Physicians. Critical Care Medicine 31:956-959, 2003.
71. Greenfield, L.J. Doctors and Nurses: A Troubled Partnership. Annals of Surgery 230:279-288, 1999.

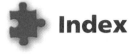

Index